The Gourmet's Companion™
Spanish
Menu Guide
&
Translator

Other Titles by Bernard Rivkin

The Gourmet's Companion: French Menu Guide & Translator
The Gourmet's Companion: German Menu Guide & Translator
The Gourmet's Companion: Italian Menu Guide & Translator

The Author wishes to express appreciation to the Spanish government tourist office for their cooperation and assistance, and the supply of some of the information used in the preparation of this book.

The Gourmet's Companion™
Spanish
Menu Guide
&
Translator

Bernard Rivkin

John Wiley & Sons, Inc.

New York • Chichester • Brisbane • Toronto • Singapore

Copyright © 1991 by Bernard Rivkin of Bellaire Publishing
Published by John Wiley & Sons, Inc.

Library of Congress Cataloging-in-Publication Data

Rivkin, Bernard.
    The gourmet's companion: Spanish menu guide and
      translator / Bernard Rivkin.
     p. cm.
    Includes bibliographical references.
    ISBN 0-471-52517-0
    1. Food—Dictionaries. 2. Cookery, Spanish—Dictionaries.
  3. Cookery—Spain. I. Title.
  TX349.R497   1991
  641.5946'03—dc20   90-38129

Printed in the United States of America
91 92 10 9 8 7 6 5 4 3 2 1

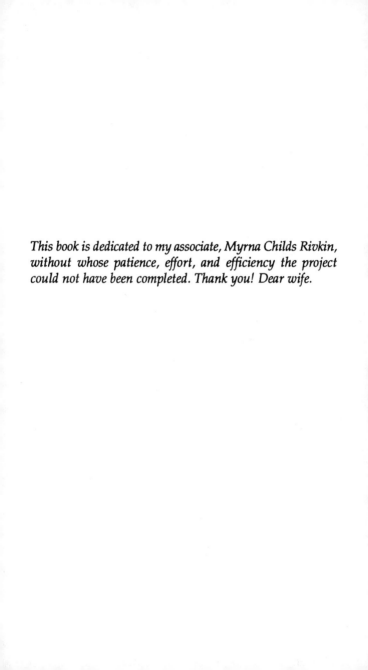

This book is dedicated to my associate, Myrna Childs Rivkin, without whose patience, effort, and efficiency the project could not have been completed. Thank you! Dear wife.

Contents

**Section 1:   Food and Drink in Spain:
               An Overview   1**

The North   2
  Galicia   3
  Asturias   5
  The Basque Country   6
  Cantabria   8
  The Ebro   9
  Aragón   9
  La Rioja   10
  Navarre   11
  Catalonia   12
    Gerona   13
    Barcelona   14
    Lérida   15
  Tarragona   16
The East Coast   17
  Castellón   17
  Alicante   18
  Valencia   19
  Murcia   21
Andalusia   22
Castile   27
  León   29
  Salamanca   29
Estremadura   30
La Mancha   32
  Madrid   34
Canary Islands   36
Balearic Islands   37

Section 2   How to Say It: English to Spanish   41

Numbers   41
Words and Phrases   42
Food and Drink   47
In the Restaurant: To Order or Make Requests   55
Problems   62
To Pay   64
Doctor/Dentist/Emergency   65
Telephone   66

Section 3:   How to Understand It: Spanish to English   69

Appetizers   69
Beverages   75
Breads   77
Cakes and Pastries   78
Cheese   81
Desserts, Fruits, and Nuts   82
Eggs   95
Fritters and Pancakes   101
Game   102
Meat   106
Potatoes   126
Poultry   127
Rice and Pasta   132
Salads   136
Sauces and Butters   140
Sausages and Pâtés   142
Seafood   145
Soups   161
Spices, Condiments, and Herbs   169

Tortillas   170
Vegetables   172
Wines, Beers, and Liquors   181

**Section 4   What It Means: A Complete
                Alphabetical Dictionary of
                Spanish Food and Drink   185**

1

Food and Drink in Spain: An Overview

Spanish cuisine relies strongly on oil and garlic. These basic and unmistakable ingredients which Spain shares with other Mediterranean countries are found in a wide variety of dishes.

Spanish cooking has basic popular roots. Although a well-served table is habitual, without making any fuss about it—except in the Basque Country and Catalonia—any refined palate without prejudices will live through some unforgettable experiences.

In this country the traveller will also discover that customs and dining habits vary considerably from one region to the next. What a difference there is between the attention, ceremony and eating capacity displayed by a *tripasai* (the term used to describe a gourmet in the Basque Country) at lunch time and the carefree, informal and casual Andalusian before a plate of fried fish.

In order to describe Spanish cooking, therefore, we have divided the peninsula into six areas with special food characteristics. In accordance with this division, the area of the sauces is the North. In the direction of the Pyrenees, there is the area of the *chilindrones* (a pepper and tomato accompaniment) which are served with many typical dishes of the region. The area of the *cazuelas* (stews) covers the greater part of Catalonia. The rice dishes are found along the East Coast. Fried dishes are typical of Andalusia, while the central area is famous for its roasts.

This is a useful arrangement because it is simple, perhaps too simple in fact. In this guide we have made it a point to describe a more detailed itinerary which, without entirely abandoning these broad outlines, is an attempt to provide as complete a view as possible of Spain's present-day cuisine.

Some dishes from the Spanish recipe book have become internationally famous, such as the paella or the *fabada*. Others, in a more modest way, have also become popular, such as the gazpacho, the tortilla, or the potato omelette. However, many typical and popular recipes have gone unnoticed. Often overlooked is what might be called the national dish par excellence, the only one which can be considered characteristic of the entire map of the art of cooking because it is found in every corner of the peninsula, though each area has its own particular version. We mean the *cocido, olla, pote* or *escudella*—in one word, the stew—which has all these different names.

The *cocido español*, or Spanish stew, has an almost universal formula consisting of three basic ingredients: meat, **pulses** (edible seeds of leguminous plants such as peas, beans, lentils) and vegetables, whatever is typical of the area, which are cooked slowly under a watchful eye. When it is ready, the dish is served in several courses, usually three, which are called *vuelcos*. First comes the soup, which is the broth in which everything was boiled, then the vegetables and pulses, and finally the meat. The common ingredient of all the Spanish *cocidos* is the chick-pea, the pea-like seed which the Carthaginians brought to Spain and which gives the Madrid and Andalusian stews, among others, their truly characteristic flavor. The *alubias* or white beans of the North give their stews a flavor which is just as tasty.

The North

In accordance with the traditional map of Spanish cuisine, the lands of Galicia, Asturias, the Basque Country and

Cantabria represent the area of the sauces. The common denominators of the cuisine are quality and abundance. The fish and seafood of the Cantabrian sea dominate the menus with unforgettable recipes in which the excellence of the raw material stands out with refined simplicity. The meat cannot be ignored either; this is the only area of the country where the vast pasture land remains green throughout the year. The stews are tasty and are made with *alubias*, the large, white beans, rather than chick-peas, which is the ingredient used in the rest of the peninsula.

The wines accompanying the food are mild, light and very different from the inland produce, especially cider which is made from apples. In this part of Spain, the servings are overwhelming and constitute, apart from the scenery, a major tourist attraction.

Galicia

The Galician cooking style is the most widespread in Spain due to the abundance of restaurants and taverns which the Galician people have brought to the faraway routes of emigration. The cuisine takes its ingredients from the sea as well as from the land.

Octopus is a very popular dish in Galicia, cooked *a fiera* (cooked whole and then cut into pieces after beating to soften it), the way it is done on the *romerías*, the festive-religious excursions to a Saint's shrine. It is seasoned with oil, paprika and salt. The *empanada* or crusted pie is symbolic of Galicia. It may be filled with an endless variety of different meats and fishes as well as a lot of onion, all of which is placed between two thin layers of oily saffron-colored pastry so that the latter does not become dry.

However, the most solemn and famous dish offered to the visitor of Galicia is *lacón con grelos* (salted ham with turnip tops). *Lacón* is pork from the cooked front leg and *grelos* are the budding top leaves of small turnips. These elements are boiled and served together with a *chorizo*, the piquant Spanish sausage, and potatoes called *cachelos*. It tastes slightly bitter and it is certainly unmistakable because of the vegetable.

Caldo gallego is an everyday dish for the Galicians. It is wonderful to eat on cold, damp days and consists of cabbage, potatoes, beans and, depending on the cook's purse, ham, chorizo, spare ribs, etc. Galicia even supplies the capital of the country with seafood and has been exporting abroad for centuries. La Coruña and Vigo, and more specifically, the village of El Grove, are a paradise where oysters, sea spiders, goose barnacles, clams and lobsters abound and can be enjoyed, *boiled and at reasonable prices.*

Special mention must be made of a very typical dish, the *vieira* or scallop served in its shell (the pilgrims who went to Compostela wore this on their cloaks). It is prepared by chopping the contents of the shell and mixing it with pepper, onions, parsley and bread crumbs. Then it is put into the oven.

As far as meat is concerned, beef is excellent, while the fattened chickens from *Villalba* are a veritable institution. They are fattened with wheat, wine and chestnuts. And for dessert, the Galicians are very fond of sweets and enjoy the following: fruit-covered cakes (which are called Episcopal cakes), almond cakes like the one called *Santiago, filoas,* a kind of sweet pancake, and *rosquillas* (biscuits).

Galicia has a very typical kind of wine, the *Ribeiro,* which must really be enjoyed in the region because it does not travel well. *Ribeiro* is served in porcelain cups and is slightly sour. Above what is typical, there is the quality wine called *Albarino,* an excellent white which comes from vines initially brought by monks from the Rhine and Moselle.

The land produces liqueurs and *eau-de-vie* which are used to prepare the most popular drink in the area: the *Queimada.* The Galicians drink the *Queimada* in the company of friends. It is prepared on the spot with *orujo* (a kind of Galician brandy made from the dregs of grapes), lemon, and sugar and then set on fire.

Among the cheeses produced in the region, the *San Simón* or *Perilla* cheese is outstanding. It is strong and smoked. The *Tetilla* is made with cow's milk, has a thin crust and a mild flavor.

Asturias

Few are the places in Spain where the traveler can eat as well and where so little fuss is made about the exquisite quality of the food. In fact, one of the most universal dishes of Spanish cuisine comes from here: the famous *fabada*, which is so successful that it is tinned and exported to all parts of America.

Fabada is genuinely Asturian and is hard to imitate. It consists of white beans called *fabes* in the region, which are especially large and soft, and different pork products: cured and salted ham bones, bacon, pig's trotters and ears, *longaniza*, a sausage, and *morcilla*, black pudding. The touch of genius in this glorious stew are the *fabes*, after which this dish is named, and the fry, wrinkled Asturian *morcilla* which miraculously comes to life in the *fabada*. It is a one-course meal served in huge quantities, which also goes for all the other dishes on the North of Spain.

Apart from the extraordinary *fabada*, Asturias has other stews in which the peerless *fabes* are a major ingredient and which the traveller should not miss. There are the delicious *fabes* with clams, hare or partridge. All these dishes are typical, though of more recent origin.

The fish dishes are based on some really tasty recipes in Asturias with mild and unmistakable flavor. At the top of the list, there is the *caldereta*, a combination of seafood and fish in a harmonious mixture. In the towns and villages of the coast this dish is prepared best, although it is not as easy to find as the *fabada*, which is served in almost every restaurant.

Hake in cider, *merluza a la sidra*, on the other hand, can be found with relative ease. Its secret lies in the quality of the raw material: the exquisite hake (a fish in the cod family) and its accompaniment, the cider, the typical drink of Asturias, made from apples. The ideal companion at the table in Asturias is the light, sour cider, which is also the most popular drink in the local bars. Drinking it is almost a ritual because it must be served by raising the bottle high and letting the liquid drop slowly into the glass without spilling a drop.

And in order to round off the itinerary along the Asturian coast, there are different ways of preparing tuna fish (*bonito*) (in dishes like *ventresca, royo, marmita*) and then there is the great star of the cuisine: the salmon. Asturias is the largest salmon-producing region in Spain. The Rivers Nalon and Sella are the most important for salmon fishing, while the classic recipe with which this specialty is prepared in Asturias is the one in which the salmon is soaked in milk, salt and lemon before grilling.

At dessert time in this region, there is no avoiding the local rice pudding, which claims to be the best in the whole of Spain and has a layer of toasted sugar on top. Apart from the rice pudding, there is a great variety of sweets such as *tocinillo de cielo* (a sweet made with egg yolk and sugar), *fayules, tortas* (flat cakes) and *bollos* (cakes). The strongest Spanish cheese, perhaps stronger than any other foreign cheese, is found here: the famous *Cabrales*, which has been compared with the French Roquefort in appearance but not in flavor.

The Basque Country

The Basque cuisine ranks first in the national cuisine despite the fact that its fame is relatively recent, but no one will argue that it is a gourmet's paradise.

It is rare to find a Basque who is not an expert regarding the cuisine. The passion, care and eating capacity of the Basques at the table are proverbial. There is no time limit to waiting nor is an occasion for it ever passed up. Institutionalized are the *amerretaco* or lunch at ten in the morning, the *amaicataco*, lunch at eleven, and the *apalaurreaudiak*, which is a tremendous tea-time-cum-dinner meal. The first societies of gastronomy in the country were also founded here.

It is a traditional cuisine which has been improved by refinements of urban and of modern origin.

Among these dishes the humble cod (*bacalao*) takes first place. Like so many other great dishes of the peninsula, *bacalao a la vizcaína* is a miracle because of the few ingredients required. It contains only cod, dried peppers and onions. The same can be said for *bacalao al pil-pil* which is cod fried with garlic and oil until the gelatine of the fish is released and turned into a delicious jelly. That jelly and the sauce with it are one of the greatest discoveries of the Basque cuisine. It is used with many other fish dishes.

Other famous sauces of this land are *la salsa verde* (green sauce) to accompany hake and the black ink based sauce which is served with squid.

Apart from cod, there is hake for which the Basques have different names depending on its size and origin. As with many other Basque food products, there is strong local competition between Guipuzcoa and Vizcaya when a decision is required about where the best hake comes from. The truth is that the rest of Spain has no equal compared with either region, be it *al pil-pil*, in a green sauce or simply fried or dipped in batter.

A refined delicacy is prepared with the small barbels of this fish. The dish is called *kokotxas* and is perhaps the tastiest of all hake dishes.

Sea bream, *besugo*, comes next. It is served grilled, cut in half and prepared with a slight touch of oil and garlic. Among the luxuries of this cuisine, there is baby eel, *angulas*, briefly dipped in boiling oil with garlic and piquant red pepper and then eaten with a wooden fork.

Of a more popular type are *el marmitako*, a tuna fish and potato stew, and the sardines, which are a symbol of the north of Spain. There the sardines are roasted as they are brought in from the sea, preferably in the month of August when they are smallest and at their tastiest. Eating sardines requires courage. Their flavor is strong, and they should be eaten using one's fingers, outdoors of course, where the fresh air will take away their smell which may otherwise cling to one's clothes.

And after this itinerary along the coast which is exclusively concerned with fish, it is time to come out in praise of the different types of meat, which are of excellent quality and are generally served roasted in huge portions. The Berritz chops are famous, and there are poultry dishes of course, which are varied but not as typical.

The only chapter in which the Basques lag behind is the one concerning wines. *Cacholi* is the only one typical of the region and it is not really very appropriate to accompany such a lavish cuisine; consequently, one would drink wines from other regions.

Idiazabal holds a place of honor among the cheeses. It is a strong cheese made from goat's milk and has a smoky flavor. As for sweet dishes, this is not really the land of people with a sweet tooth, but typical are the stuffed Vergara biscuits, *Bilbao canutillos*, and pears prepared in the oven.

Cantabria

It is very difficult to define the cuisine here clearly because it consists of what has come from the surrounding areas, with which it shares the raw materials. This is a region which has absorbed many if the Castilian cooking habits. It is a place where one can eat very well, which is true everywhere in the North. Here again we find tuna, hake, sea bream and salmon, which is prepared in an absolutely unique fashion: *el arroz santanderino*, which is rice with salmon and milk. There are also sardines and anchovies, the latter either in a stew or crusted pie, in a yellow sauce or in a batter. Another typical dish consists of *rabas*, which is squid chopped up and fried.

However, it is in the chapter of desserts where the cuisine of Santander offers the most original dishes: custard, which is extraordinary thanks to the natural flavor of the ingredients, only milk and eggs; and *los sobaos pasiegos*, pastry rich in butter and eggs. Both of these are at the top of the list, together with *la quesada*, one of the most popular of the national sweets, made with fresh cheese, honey and butter, the only problem being the limited time for which it can be kept.

The Ebro

This is a region with a very characteristic cuisine around the Ebro river which is commonly known as the one of the *chilindrones* (a sauce made with pepper, tomato and fried onion). However the description is only partly appropriate. This is a region of very good food, which is hearty and plentiful. There are also the wines, the Rioja, though there are some less-known varieties, such as the stronger Cariñena wines. The production of meat products is flourishing, especially *longaniza* (a sausage) and ham.

Aragón

This region is famous for one of the most straightforward cuisines in Spain.

Meat is the basis of Aragonese cuisine and *chilindrón*, its most typical formula. Chicken, lamb and pork are all found in this sauce as easily as other meat, though it is most commonly prepared with chicken, In the Upper Aragón region, in the heart of the mountains, more rustic cooking is popular: lamb and goat roasted on the spit, lamb and vegetable stew (*a la pastora*) and the so-called *espárragos montañeses* (literally, "mountain asparagus"), which are in fact calves' tails.

On the way to Saragossa, *las magras con tomate* are overwhelmingly tasty: slices of slightly fried ham dipped in tomato sauce. Then there is an endless variety accompanying *las migas*, a dish which has become very popular everywhere in the central area of the peninsula. But nowhere is it served in so many varieties. Here they are served with croutons—of ham, *chorizo*, bacon, black pudding, with chocolate and grapes. And they are always made with good bread, cut into small pieces and prepared with the chosen accompaniment. In some places they are soaked in water or milk before being fried.

More exquisite recipes include partridge with chocolate, which has become popular throughout the country; fried trout from the Pyrenees which are of the best quality in those rivers; and the tasty hams of Teruel, which are cured in the cruel winter cold of its mountains. Let's not forget the soups, like the one with liver and cheese, which was already mentioned in the 17th century as *sopa aragonese*. It is prepared in the oven with slices of toasted bread.

Among the vegetables, there is one which is exclusive to the Moncayo region: borage which is tastier than beet or spinach, but distantly related to the same family. Vegetable stew, *menestra*, is prepared with the rich produce of the region.

Among typical exotic dishes, there is a well-liked dish that must not be forgotten: baked lamb's head; as well as the humble invention of the *reganaos*, which consist of pastry with a couple of sardines and a few strips of red pepper in the crust.

Aragonese wines are as abundant as they are good. In any bar or tavern, you will be sure to find exceptional examples. The only wine which is known at a national level is the *Cariñena*, which has an alcohol content of 18 percent.

Among the desserts, pears in wine should be tried as well as Aragonese candied or chocolate-covered fruit, and two almond pastes, *guirlache* and *turrón*.

La Rioja

In this region, the first topic is the wine, which has become famous far beyond the Spanish borders. Rioja wine has a very long history and the first documents about it date back to the 17th century. In many cases they are still made with the old traditional methods and in the same old wineries. The Rioja wines are basically red to light red, have a great bouquet, a mild taste and a moderate alcohol content, which is between 12 and 14 percent.

The cuisine of the area, which is not as well-known as its wines, has its own style called *a la riojana* (in the style of La Rioja), with which different meat, poultry and vegetables are prepared. It consists of a fried mixture of red pepper, *chorizo* and asparagus.

A really exclusive dish (though it is poorly imitated in many areas) consists of stuffed peppers which will prove to be an exquisite discovery: the delicious red peppers of the region filled with chopped pork and bread crumbs.

In the Rioja, meat is also very good (roasted chops, chicken, sirloin with peppers) and so are vegetables (either stewed, fried or mixed and cooked), the most outstanding being asparagus and pepper. Apart from the cuisine as such, there is the joy, without stiff-necked ceremony or boredom, connected with the local customs that are followed in these parts when it comes to eating and drinking.

Navarre

The cuisine in this area is eclectic and shares its tastes with different sources: the Basque, French and Aragonese cuisine. It has a wide range, is well-stocked and will not disappoint the visitor with some of its best recipes: *la trucha a la navarra* (trout fried with a piece of ham), which has become popular everywhere in Spain as a masterly formula for preparing this fish. However, nowhere is it better than here where it has its origin. First the fish is soaked in wine, then it is filled with a slice of ham and dipped in flour before frying.

Regarding meat, there are lamb chops and *el cochifrito navarro* (small pieces of fried lamb). Among the stews, there is a vegetable soup which is very similar to a soup called *garbure* in France. It is a dish for green vegetable lovers because it consists of beet greens, spinach, mallow, sorrel and lettuce.

Dishes of feathered game deserve special mention in Navarre, since they are especially well-liked by the people of Navarre and they do not abound in the present Spanish cuisine, more than anything because of the absence of the main ingredient. Bird shooting is a very popular activity in Navarre: quail, turtledove and wood pigeon in particular.

With all of these birds exquisite dishes are prepared. Quail is fattest in the month of September, and is roasted in fig leaves. Turtledove is roasted with herbs on the grill, covered with oil, lard, vinegar and red wine. Partridge is also prepared in accordance with old recipes with a chocolate sauce. This sauce also accompanies hare and rabbit. These dishes are not common and are usually prepared and served on special occasions.

The picture of the cuisine of the area is not complete without the *roncal* cheese, which is among the best in the country, and *la chistorra*, a very characteristic sausage, prepared over burning charcoal and served with a drink before lunch or in the afternoon.

Catalonia

Of all the regional cuisines in the peninsula, Catalán cooking is without a doubt the most sophisticated, complete and richest—apart from possessing the most historical evidence. It is, in short, a privileged cuisine, because it developed at crossroads that have connected it throughout history with many other countries, such as France and Italy.

Its main dishes rely on four basic sauces: *sofrito*, *samfaina*, *picada* and *alioli*, and of the four, special mention must be made of the second, because it is strictly Catalán and used with a wide variety of dishes. It is a half-cooked mixture of tomato, pepper and eggplant. *Sofrito*, on the other hand, is rather widespread in Spanish cooking. It is a fried sauce made with garlic, onion, tomato and parsley. *Picada* has the special Catalán touch and is added to the simplest dishes so that they never become monotonous routine. It contains garlic, parsley, toasted almonds and chopped pine seeds. *Alioli* is an admirable dressing which probably dates from the time of the Romans and is made with olive oil and garlic which are mixed very patiently in the mortar until they turn into a creamy paste which is ideal for meat and fish.

The traveler will discover a variety of rice dishes in Catalonia, as well as meat dishes, particularly poultry, and the famous Gerona veal; not to mention the rock fish, which is prepared very tastily and with a lot of imagination. The visitor will also find a surprisingly rich collection of sausages, including *butifarra* which is roasted or fried with *monjetes* (white beans) to make a modest but tasty dish, and one of the most typical in the region. Accompanying this dish is another very traditional treat: bread with tomato, in a Catalán version, a sandwich which is much juicier than anywhere else. The bread is first covered with oil, tomato and salt, and then a slice of cured ham, an omelette or whatever is at hand may be put on top.

The wines in the area are also magnificent. Worthy of special mention are those of *El Priorato*, which are very special, thick and mild reds not readily found outside Catalonia. *El porrón* or glass jug is also very popular in Catalonia: the wine is poured from the glass jug with the spout held high. More common is the leather wineskin, which is equally appropriate for the liquid, but drinking from the *porrón* seems to give the wine a different taste.

Gerona

Of all Catalonia, Gerona really has the best cuisine. It covers part of the Pyrenees and part of the Mediterranean and has carefully preserved its cooking traditions. The area inland, Ampurdan, has the best dishes of feathered animals. It is the area of the largest turkeys, geese, ducks and poultry stuffed with complicated and unforgettable mixtures of pears, turnips, apples, and olives. It is also especially famous for its Christmas turkey, stuffed with sausages, *butifarras*, raisins and pine nuts. Game also abounds on the recipes: rabbits are prepared with fine herbs, hare with chestnuts, partridge in accordance with a recipe originating from Olesa. Here we find a cuisine which likes to mix flavors, sweet and salty or fish and meat. In this sense, it may be said that it has the most unusual dish of all Spanish cuisine, which is nevertheless magnificent: the little-known *Mar y cielo* ("sea and heaven"), which contains nothing less than sausages, rabbit, shrimp and angler and is prepared in Estartit. And finally there is another famous Costa Brava dish: chicken with lobster.

In the chapter about fish, Gerona, with the rest of the Costa Brava, stands out among all the Catalán areas for its magnificent *suquets*, a fisherman's dish which contains different rockfish boiled in a thick broth and an equally thick *sofrito*. The thick and magnificent angler soup must also be mentioned, and the lobster which is the best in the region and is prepared with roasted almonds and garlic and then served with *alioli*.

Finally there are the meat products. Vic is the capital of the sausage called *salchichón* in Catalonia's special version known as *fuett*, and of the *butifarra* which is also exclusive and prepared in a thousand different ways: made with blood, raw, cooked, spicy, with eggs.

Barcelona

Barcelona is a city which has a long tradition in the art of cooking. It reached its greatest splendor in this sense in the 19th century, when some of its many restaurants were counted among the best in Europe.

Of the most important dishes, special mention should be made of the *escudella i carn d'olla*, which was eaten almost daily until the thirties. Today it can hardly be found in the local restaurants. However, it is still number one of the typical Catalán dishes.

Escudella is the Catalán version of the chick-pea stew called *cocido*. It is based on the same principle of cooking meat and vegetables together. There are two separate courses, that is, two dishes: one, a soup with small noodles and rice, and then meat, served with the vegetables. It does not include *chorizo* or *morcilla* like other Spanish stews, but the white and black *butifarra* and the famous *pilota*, a ball made of meat, parsley, bread crumbs and egg. This stew probably has more ingredients than any other stew in the whole country: beef, hen, bacon, pig's ear, pig's trotters and lean pork, white and black *butifarra*, ham bone, marrow bone, chick-peas, beans, potatoes, cauliflower, egg, turnip, carrot, garlic, flour, pepper, cinnamon and parsley.

The people of Barcelona have also invented tasty noodles, which are called *fideos a la cazuela*, one of the most popular dishes of the region. As is customary in this area, the dish includes an ample selection of spare ribs, sausages, *butifarra*, ham and bacon as well as *sofrito* which, as usual, consists of onion, pepper and tomato.

Together with the *escudella* and *butifarra* with beans, which we mentioned in the introduction, the third most typical Catalán stew is the one with broad beans (*habas a la catalana*). It is prepared with a lot of herbs and spices (thyme, rosemary, mint, cinnamon and bay leaf), broad beans (which are the favorite vegetable in the area) and *butifarra*.

As for desserts, Catalán cream is excellent. It resembles custard and is covered with a layer of caramel. However, the most traditional sweets are the ones prepared all through the year for the different holidays, such as *pan de pesic, las cocas de la noche de San Juan, los panallets* of almonds and pine seeds in the month of November, and at any time of the year, *el mel i mato* with *requesón*, a soft, white cheese.

Lérida

Lérida cooking resembles the hearty mountain cuisine, in which game and excellent trout abound. In order to enjoy them at their best, one should select one of the little food-serving places on the Pyrenees, with an expert cook. And reserve the meal in advance. Thus, there is a chance of trying *la cassolada,* a potato-and-vegetable stew with bacon and ribs; or lamb's head and legs with *girella,* or lamb's feet with turnips, and above all, the excellent hare and chamois *civets.*

In this region rice dishes are frequently prepared with rabbit, cod and pork. They are always served with a lot of broth. The most typical sausages of the region are *la girella* and *los xolis.*

Tarragona

This province is noted for such dishes as rabbit with garlic and tuna boiled with potatoes, *pataca* (Jerusalem artichoke), marrow and snails, balls of cod and cod fritters. There is also a great specialty, *los calcots* which are sweet, tender onions, the shoots of an old onion. This dish is served in Alls and throughout the area around Poblet and Santa Creus under the name of *calcotada.* It is a typical and exotic dish: the onions, freshly picked, are roasted and served on a tile, accompanied by an olive oil and almond sauce.

However, most important of the Tarragona cuisine are the rice dishes and a really splendid sauce. Among the rice dishes, *el arrosext* is a particularly popular one along the East Coast and is especially typical of fishermen. Then there is the black rice with sepia and *el arroz abanda,* the most extraordinary of all the rice dishes in Spanish cuisine. However, it should be eaten only in absolutely reliable places. In Tarragona, by way of Cambrils, the best are served without any doubt.

Arroz abanda is a rice dish meant for experts because it is served by itself, or, if one wants, together with the fish with which it was boiled. The fish and seafood must be of the best quality and the greatest possible variety: grouper, angler, conger, prawns, lobster and squid. The complete dish consists of a large amount of rice, which has been boiled with all the fish, and another dish of fish which is served with *alioli* or *romesco*.

Romesco is very popular along the Mediterranean coast and has become part of international cuisine. Experts do not agree on the ideal formula or on its variations. Some say olive oil, red pepper and bread are enough, while others add garlic, almonds, cognac, vinegar, and then cook it all. Whatever the case, *romesco* is the name of a special red pepper used in its preparation, and together with *alioli* it is the most typical of the Mediterranean sauces.

The Priorato wines are the product of the Tarragona vineyards. They are excellent reds. some with 14 percent and others with up to 20 percent. The higher-lying areas are justly famous for the sparkling wines or *cavas* of San Sadurni de Noya.

The East Coast

It is not at all difficult to describe the main ingredient if the cuisine of this area: it is the kingdom of rice.

The native of Valencia has learned to control this very modest element to perfection and obtains the most exquisite results, whether the cook adds a veritable army of ingredients or practically nothing.

And here we find one of the most universal dishes of the Spanish cuisine *la paella*. which is a masterpiece of the art of cooking. However, it has become so widespread that at times it is almost unrecognizable.

Castellón

Around the Maestrazgo inland this province offers meat dishes, lamb, and heavy stews, based on potato, corn, flour, almonds and walnuts. Baked kid goat, larded meat and tripe are prepared, as are stews or *ollas*. The famous Castellón *olla* can be found everywhere in the province.

It is prepared with white beans, beef and bacon. However, perhaps the most typical dishes are those made with rice: rice with green beans and snails and the famous *arroz empedrado*, which contains tomatoes and cod and a top layer of white beans. *Arroz a la marinera* is served all along the coast, and if we approach the sea, we should, if possible, try the prawns which are really excellent.

Fine cheeses are also made in Satellón, though they do not usually travel beyond its borders. *La colla*, a type of yogurt made with the pistils of wild artichokes, deserves special mention. Some of the popular local sweets are *mostatxones* and *las puntas de diamante*.

Alicante

Here the recipes of La Mancha, Valencia and Murcia can all be found, and it is not very easy to find the most original dishes in public places. There are, for example, the *paella alicantina*, which has no seafood, only chicken and rabbit, and *los bajoques farcides*, which are peppers stuffed with rice, pork, tomatoes and spices; the vegetable stews with rice, potatoes and beans, and *la pericana*, a winter dish made during the olive harvest to test the quality of the olives. It contains cod, oil, dry peppers and garlic.

To honor a guest or celebrate a special festive occasion, there is the original and tasty *cocido de pelotas* (a stew whose main ingredient is minced meat wrapped in cabbage leaves apart from chicken or turkey, lean pork bacon, chick-peas, potatoes and spices).

In Elche, the town of palm trees, a very original kind of rice dish is preserved like a treasure. This family recipe is laborious and delicate: *arroz con costra*, which has conquered the whole of the East Coast, though its origin and best version is found here. It contains a huge number of ingredients: chicken, rabbit, sausages, black pudding, chick-peas and spices, and on top of all this, meatballs made of pork and bread crumbs. All this is then "hidden" under beaten egg and put in the oven to form a delicious crust.

Alicante really takes the spotlight when it comes to desserts, for the area has excellent dates which are sold everywhere in Spain, and another very old fruit, the pomegranate. However, *el turrón* (almond paste) has really made the name of Alicante universal when it comes to sweets.

It is fairly safe to say that this sweet is of Arab origin. *El turrón* made in Alicante is of two types: the one which carries its name is made from whole almonds in a mass of honey and sugar; and the one of Jijona, in which the almond is ground. There are others of the soft type, with flavors such as chocolate, fruit, and coconut. They are more modern and have nothing to do with the traditional almond paste or *turrón*.

Valencia

Although Valencia used to be famous for its excellent food in the 15th century, today the cuisine of Valencia means above all and almost exclusively *paella*.

La paella is of recent origin, that is, the middle of the 19th century, and it was first prepared in the region of La Albufera outside Valencia.

The secret of the *paella*, as well as of the other rice dishes of Valencia, lies in the unique texture of the grain after cooking. The grain is loose, dry and soft at the same time. The next priority is the flavor from the huge range of ingredients which puts a stop to any conversation about the austerity of Spanish cooking.

This famous and most representative Spanish dish really has no specific recipe. In any case, a good *paella* may easily include chicken, pork, shellfish, eel, squid, beans, peas, artichokes and fresh peppers. In addition, the secret ingredient must not be forgotten: saffron, which is also used for rice in Milan and Marseille.

After the splendid *paella*, there is an endless number of rice dishes parading through the cuisine of Valencia, with varying accompaniments, especially *el arroz amb frejol i nabo* (rice with beans and turnips), which until recently was considered the daily fare of the farmers and which is rather soupy. A variety of the same dish includes pig's trotters, pig's ears and black pudding. Then there is the so-called *arroz en oros y bastos*, a name referring to the figures on Spanish playing cards.

There are also special rice dishes for the days of fasting. These are prepared with kidney beans and potatoes, others with snails and spinach, or small squid and cauliflower, or chick-peas and a couple of slices of tomato. The list would be endless, but a few more of the classical rice dishes deserve to be mentioned: *arroz a la Alcirena*, which is done in the oven and is very similar to the one of Elche, and *el arroz rosetxat*, which is also put in the oven.

Besides the forceful attraction of the rice dishes in the cuisine of Valencia, there are different fish dishes, seasoned with *alipebre*, a garlic, olive oil and paprika sauce, which is very popular in the region. This sauce is served with eels, which are prepared on the grill or roasted over ash wood. Red mullet and sepia are very popular. The Albufera duck had a very good name, and although there aren't any today, many delicious recipes still survive, among them, *el pato a la naranja* (duck and orange), which is a very old Valencian dish.

For dessert, the people of Valencia have a lot to offer, especially on festive-religious occasions. There are roasted almonds, toasted bread, Easter buns (*monas*), *arnadi* (made of gourd and sugared chestnuts), *suspiros*, egg rolls and an endless series of cookies and cakes.

There is also a huge variety of white wines in Valencia, light and dry ones from Albaida, Chesete and Liria and *olorosos* from the same area. The reds and light reds are from Utiel and Requena where the grape harvest is celebrated every year and a fountain is set up from which wine flows free of charge. A visit to Valencia would be incomplete without mentioning another very popular local drink, *horchata*, made from *chufas* or earth almonds. It is a light, sweet and refreshing drink which is popular as a summer beverage everywhere in Spain.

Murcia

The cuisine of Murcia is one of the most typical and well-preserved in Spain and one of the least known. It is a cuisine of the East Coast which relies on the products of the orchard and a secret Arab influence. Fresh pepper and tomato are preferred and used in an entirely different way compared with Aragón or La Rioja.

As for rice dishes, there are many and there are those who say that the ones in Murcia are better than the ones in Valencia. They are prepared with chicken, rabbit, *mujol* (which is a local fish, the roe of which is exquisite and a very common specialty) and all kinds of vegetables. Another delicious rice dish is *el arroz al caldero*, made with local fish.

The people of Murcia can be proud of their excellent vegetables. The vegetable stew called *menestra* is magnificent. So are the artichokes fried with tomatoes, pickles, eggplant, cauliflower boiled or in béchamel. And above all, *los michirones*, which are beans served either in an omelette, stewed or uncooked with a salad dressing.

Omelettes are served in a variety of ways. Apart from the one with beans, there are omelettes with garlic shoots or pepper and tomato. Scrambled eggs come with asparagus and in a endless variety of combinations. The local produce is of such excellent quality that the lettuce, which is prepared by cutting the center into four portions, dressed with olive oil, lemon and pepper, is called the "Orchard Partridge."

Apart from the orchard lands, there are fish dishes that are a real luxury, like the prawns from the Mar menor, which are small and extremely tasty; the already mentioned roe of the *mujol*, which is worth its weight in gold; and the more popular sea bass coated with salt and put in the oven.

There are also stews and vegetable dishes typical of the East Coast as well as meat recipes with lamb, chicken and rabbit, which are often served with tomatoes and peppers.

Among the meat dishes, special mention should be made of the meat pie, made with veal, *chorizo*, hard-boiled egg, brains and minced meat, all wrapped in a fine layer of pastry and baked in the oven. It is a lovely old dish which is served on special occasions, the more modern version of which is *el Pastel de Cierva*.

Murcia has a very typical series of meat products, including *longaniza* and black pudding, which are very mild and spiced and have an exquisite taste.

The sweet dishes are of Arab origin like those from Valencia. There is even one called Allah's Bread (*pan de Alá*), besides fig bread, walnut cakes, *tocino de cielo*, *roscos de vino* and the famous marmalades and syrups.

The chapter on wines has two parts: one on the Jumilla wines, which are among the strongest in the country, and one on the peerless rosés and light reds, which are, together with those from Cigales in Valladolid, the best in the country.

Andalusia

Andalusia which, from the point of view of cooking, comes under the heading of fried food, has a rich and traditional cuisine, which cannot be said of all of its nine provinces and which the traveler may not find easily.

The best wines of Spain come from Andalusia and belong to the long list of Spanish wines which are most famous abroad. The wines of Jerez in the Province of Cádiz are the most renowned in universal literature, beginning with Greek texts of the 4th century B.C.

The system of production is unique and almost borders on the miraculous, for it is not a wine from a specific crop, as is the custom in other places, but from successive mixtures made over the years.

These are wines that must be sipped slowly. and savored in the course of a conversation with or without a *tapa* (an appetizer).

And after the wines, the ham. The best ham in the country is produced in Andalusia: the *Jabugo* in Huelva. It is unique and definitely superior to any other in the peninsula, although the ham from Trevelez on Granada is almost as good. Both should be cut in fine slices as opposed to Castilian hams which are best served in small cubes.

Then there is the famous *pescaito frito* (deep-fried fish), which has two main capitals: Cádiz and Málaga, though it is prepared everywhere in Andalusia.

In Cádiz, the fish is sold to the public in fish shops or at stalls, and it is impossible to give a definite recipe for their preparation. It may be the way the fish is cut, the temperature of the olive oil used to fry it or the special aroma which is produced by frying different species of fish together in the same pan: *mojarras* (Diplodus vulgaris), sole, gray and red mullet, whiting.

In Málaga, fried fish is a different, but equally delicious treat. There, *el boquerón* (fresh baby anchovy) is king. It is fried in huge piles and put on the plate where it resembles the "foam in the sea," as the tiny *chanquetes* (baby anchovies just born) have been called. Fried fish is also found in Seville though there it is prepared in larger pieces and dipped in a special pastry called *adobo*.

Another typical aspect of Andalusian cooking is *el gazpacho*, a favorite dish in the Spanish summer. It is a soup which is prepared in a thousand different ways, though Córdoba probably makes the best. It consists of bread, oil, garlic and water and very often tomato. There is no reason why fresh pepper and cucumber should not be added, though they are not traditional.

Among the splendid variations, there is the *Salmorejo* of Córdoba, one of the traditional dishes which has managed to survive in the province. It is, like all Anadalusian gazpachos, a cold dish which consists of tomato, bread, olive oil, garlic and pepper and is served in the shape of a very hearty soup. Special mention should be made of the typical gazpacho of Málaga called *ajo blanco*, which is less common than the Andalusian version, but is equally refreshing and much more original. It is made with oil, almonds and garlic and patiently prepared in the mortar until it becomes a paste to which cold water is added. The final touch is provided by a few grapes.

Regarding heartier dishes, the province of Cádiz comes first. Its cuisine is without a doubt the richest and most varied in Andalusia. In addition to the *pescaito frito* and the best shellfish and mollusks along the coast (*el ostión* or giant oyster, prawn, shrimp, small clam, crab), there are kidneys in sherry, pigeon pie, oxtail and squid with beans. There is also a very popular and typical old stew with a proud name and unheard-of-taste: *el caldillo de perro* (literally, dog soup).

It is prepared in the local taverns where the fishermen live, and the outcome, half salty, half sour, is not at all easy to predict despite its few ingredients. It contains onions, fresh fish and orange juice.

Of the famous recipes of the Andalusian cuisine, dishes from Granada, the great cuisine area, are outstanding: *las habas a la granadina* and *la tortolla Sacromonte*. The former includes Trevelez ham and *el ramillete albaicinero*, a bunch of herbs from the Sierra of El Albaicín including bay leaf, mint and parsley. This recipe, together with those of Catalonia, are the best ones for beans.

La tortilla Sacromonte is a festive omelette of extraordinary refinement which should never be mistaken for the so-called *paisana* which abounds on the menus of restaurants. The Sacromonte omelette is made with fried and breaded brain, lamb or veal testicles, potatoes, red pepper and peas. Everything is cut into small pieces and sautéed before adding the eggs. As a dish it is almost a ritual, closely linked to the gypsy cave dwellings in Sacromonte, after which it is called. The Granada *tortilla* is a variation of this omelette, but it is made with lamb sweetbreads, chicken liver and kidney with white wine.

Another important Granada dish is a noodle dish called *cazuela de fideos* with beans and cod and a whole range of spices. Along the coast around Motril and Almuñécar, the popular *moragas de sardinas* (fresh anchovies on a spit) are prepared. This fish is spitted whole, the stick is stuck into the sand and hot embers are arranged around it to roast the fish.

In Almería, the cuisine is partly from Murcia and partly from Granada. The same can be said of another border province, Jaén. There the typical dishes are partly from La Mancha, Granada and Córdoba. Spinach is part of one of the most popular dishes of Jaén when served with crushed dried peppers, garlic bread crust, and plenty of olive oil. Since Jaén produces most of the olive oil that comes from Spain, this oil is used freely with salads as in the *pipirrana*, a mixture of green pepper, onion, tomato and marinated fish in small pieces.

In Córdoba the traditional recipes have largely been forgotten. Oxtail stew, which is strong, greasy and very tasty, though reminiscent of bullfighting, has recently become the top regional dish. There are also gazpachos as described, and veal with artichokes, pigeons with olives and baked pig's trotters. Worthy of special mention are the wines in this province which have their own unique taste, capable of competing with their famous neighbor, Jerez. The wines are dry, fragrant and have a high alcohol content. They have an official Certificate of Origin (*Appellation d'origine*): Moriles-Montilla, and there are four types: finos, amontillados, *olorosos* and aged *oloroses*. The best wines are those which come from the Montilla mountains, the so-called Montilla Albero and Moriles Albero.

Another province which does not lag behind in terms of wines is Málaga with its famous *moscatel*, one of the best Spanish productions. It comes from the grape of the same name, perhaps the most exquisite in the world. Málaga wine resembles liqueur, has a warm taste and a dark color. It is sold under many different names; including *Málaga*, *Málaga Virgen*, *Lacrima Christi*, and *Pedro Ximénez*.

Apart from the Jabugo ham, which is glory enough in itself, Huelva has some splendid fish dishes: red bream with onions, sardines with black pepper, red bream in paprika, clams with rice and *chocos* (squid-like fish, typical along this coast, which are very tasty) in different recipes.

Finally, there is Seville, the official capital of these lands. This is the kingdom of the *tapa*, a delicious, small-scale hors d'oeuvre which has successfully found its way into every corner of the country. But no imitation has come close to the mastery of Seville on scope and variety of its ingredients.

The traveller who passes the test of the *tapas* in Seville will discover some important typical dishes, for example, the famous *huevos a la flamenca*, a simple, but elegant recipe which can now be found everywhere in Spain. Preparation of this recipe is delicate and should be served as soon as it is ready. The eggs are put in the oven on a bed of small pieces of tomatoes, *chorizo*, ham, green beans, fried potatoes, asparagus, red pepper and peas.

Another popular dish of Seville is tripe, called *menudo gitano*, *el cocido a la sevillana* (a stew), in which the meat is fried with beaten eggs, *termedra a la sevillana*, larded veal with wine and olives, and finally duck with olives.

As for sweet dishes, Andalusia has an endless variety which are of obvious Arab origin. These have been often admirably preserved by the nuns of the many convents in the area, especially in those of Seville. *Las tortas* (oil cakes), which are sold everywhere in the country, are a typical breakfast in countless cities and are made in the convents. *Los polvorones* (which are typical at Christmas), *los cortadillos*, with a pumpkin filling, *los alfajores, mostachones* (small cakes for dipping in coffee or hot chocolate) are among the traditional sweets as well as *las yemas de San Leandro* (egg yolks).

Castile

As in Andalusia, Castilian cuisine covers a considerable area. It differs from Andalusia in that it is more uniform in its fare and recipes, with the exception of two areas: León and Salamanca. The rest of the provinces in the area (Burgos, Soria, Ávila, Segovia, Zamora, Valladolid and Valencia) fit perfectly into the picture of the art of cooking that we are going to describe, an area which comes under the heading of the Land of Roasts.

In Castilian cuisine, the chick-pea is the first ingredient that comes to mind. It is the element which has presided over the food in this area for centuries, especially if we keep to the popular everyday fare of the people.

This dried vegetable, which was brought to Spain by the Carthaginians, is the main ingredient of all Castilian stews. Until fairly recently, it was the daily fare in all Spanish homes. It was always prepared with cabbage, and depending on one's finances, with black pudding, chorizo and meat.

After the chick-pea, other vegetables are important in Castilian cookery. Among them are large white beans (*alubias*) and lentils, which are prepared with chorizo, oxtail, or pig's ear and are of excellent quality like the chick-pea.

And after the vegetables, bread and wine. Bread is the symbol of Castile, "the land of bread," and is tastier there than anywhere else in Spain, though it has lost a great deal of importance as a staple food. Wine, on the other hand, has not lost any of its importance, and Castile is awash with magnificent wines. They are strong and dry and almost always red, though Rueda is noted for its whites and Cigales for its rosés. Especially outstanding are the wines grown in the province of Valladolid, around Quintanilla de Onésimo, which are world famous.

However, there is one dish which stands out from everything else in Castilian cuisine and fare, at least from the tourist point of view: the typical roast suckling pig and lamb.

The roasts are found along two itineraries in Castile. First, the itinerary of the lamb, *cordero*, forms a magic triangle with Segovia-Soria-Burgos, in which Segovia is especially important.

Castilian lamb is always roasted in a clay dish and does not require any skill other than spreading lard on it, sprinkling salted water over the skin and roasting it until it is just right.

The other itinerary of the roasts is the one of the suckling pig or *tostón*. It is best in the area limited by Segovia-Arévalo-Penaranda de Bracamonte. *El cochinillo* is a recently born pig. To comply with specifications, it must be between fifteen and twenty days old and weigh between three and four kilos. It should be roasted in an oven with thyme and must be tender enough to permit a nimble and spectacular act: the cook must be able to divide the pig into portions with the edge of a plate.

It should also be remembered that although Castile is far from the sea, it has some excellent fish dishes. One of them has become popular throughout the entire country: *bacalao al ajo arriero* (a cod and garlic dish) named after the Leonese mule drivers (*arrieros*) who took this dish to Estremadura, Andalusia, Navarre, the North and La Mancha.

In addition to cod, Castile has some splendid trout dishes. The species abounds in its rivers as does river crab, which is an exquisite dish, especially when it is served with a very tasty red sauce.The best trout are said to come from the Tormes river. But it is on the Pisuerga where a festival is held every year in honor of this animal, which becomes rarer and rarer because too many are caught.

Let us complete the list of Castilian dishes with *pepitorias de gallina* (a fricassee), rice with chicken, stuffed partridge and quail, rabbit with garlic and the very popular *sopas castellanas* which consist of bread, preferably the broth of a stew, ham, sometimes a poached egg and garlic, of course.

Garlic is the spice par excellence in Castile, and it is used as frequently as in other areas of the country, but the difference is that here its presence is much more noticeable.

In this general picture, there are two exceptions which are the cuisines of two areas that belong to Castile, geographically speaking, but have nothing to do with it when it comes to cooking: the provinces of León and Salamanca.

León

This province has a famous past going back to the Middle Ages, when the great lords of the castles and the rich monasteries of the region took their high standards of cooking beyond their borders. Today there are two major trends. One centers around the region of El Bierzo, which is reminiscent of Galician cuisine: *empanadas* or crusted pies, salted pork with turnip tops, and octopus prepared as it is in Galicia. The other is the Astorga region which is the area known as La Maragatería, where the stew called *cocido maragato*, the vegetables called *menestra de Riano* and the cod dish called *bacalao al ajo arriero* are found.

Salamanca

In this province the cuisine consists essentially of beef and game. The cuisine is solid and heavy, combining vegetables and meat to the best advantage. Its restaurants make a point of offering the traditional dishes and so it is easy to find *chanfaina salmantina*, made with rice, giblet, lamb sweetbread and pieces of *chorizo. Los farinatos* is a sausage which is fried and served with eggs. And there is also a great variety of meat stews, each with a character of its own: stewed calf's tail, stewed tongue, ragout, veal lips in batter, lamb stew, roast kid goat, and stuffed chicken.

A description of the cuisine of Castile is incomplete without the cheeses which may not be as famous as the products of La Mancha, but are not really far behind. In this region, there are creamy and cured quality cheeses, but there are also bland white cheeses which are less frequent in the rest of the country. Among these the ones from Villalonín, Valladolid, and Burgos are famous.

Among the sweets, roast almonds covered with caramel sugar are outstanding and have conquered the Spanish market from Briviesca in Burgos.

Estremadura

Pork from Estremadura is the pride of Spain. Until very recently the pig used to live on the acorns of the grazing lands and grew up wild. The best pork products came from there, and like the Montánchez ham and chorizos are prepared in a thousand different ways: sour-sweet, piquant, sweet, thick, middling, thin and roasted. Other products are larded loin, white sausage, black pudding with potatoes, and pork pâté from Mérida, with which half the country is supplied.

As far as stews are concerned, the people of Estremadura have few, but the ones they have are outstanding. There are *el frite* and *la caldereta*, which are prepared with lamb and baby goat respectively. There are also *los pucheros*, *las migas* and *las gachas* which are basic dishes, especially the first two, one from around Badajoz, while the other is more often found in Cáceres.

La caldereta consists of kid goat, cut into pieces and fried and cooked with piquant peppers and seasoned with mashed liver, raw garlic and red peppers. It is a shepherd's dish to be eaten from an iron pot which is suspended over burning branches under a holm oak. The same goes for *el frite*, which is country and excursion fare. It is prepared with pieces of a yearling lamb and fried with paprika until it turns red and leaves slight traces of olive oil on the plate.

These are festive dishes, but there are others like lamb's tail prepared in a big pot with a thick sauce which emphasizes the soft juicy texture of the tails.

And as is to be expected, pork is used for everything apart from sausages. There is minced meat, ears in batter and sauce, tail with tomato, lean meat with potatoes, *pastorejos* (slices from the head of the animal) with fried eggs, and a kind of thick heavy soup called *jcachuela* which is prepared with sweetbreads, blood, liver, and tripe of the pig. All these stews are heavy, definitely the invention of shepherds and are meant for tough stomachs and palates for which diet is an unknown word.

And without going beyond the old country cuisine, there is a singularly attractive dish: *las migas*. It is a modest one but very popular in central Spain. In Estremadura it used to be the daily fare for a long time, and there it is made with a magic touch. To begin with, bread is soaked in water and then fried with pieces of bacon and dry peppers. It is no longer an everyday dish, but if ordered in advance, it is prepared as well as ever in any restaurant.

El gazpacho extremeño consists of a soup with pieces of tomato which are not blended to a liquid consistency as are the rest of the ingredients Onion is also added, an ingredient never found in the Andalusian variety. Another dish is *sopas enganadas*, an original and strange mixture consisting of pepper, onion shoots in vinegar, figs and grapes.

Some dishes are made with fish: *el ajo de peces de río* (literally. "garlic with river fish") is typical in the area around Badajoz. It is like a *gazpacho* with fish, because it is boiled with a lot of mashed garlic. It is similar to the way gazpacho is prepared with recipes from the convents: *el recado de patatas*, with potatoes in batter and a sauce accompanying the fish, and *el bacalao del convento*, which consists of potatoes, spinach and some broth.

Frog legs are also very popular. They are fried in a batter or served in a tomato sauce.

Regarding desserts, the fruit from the Don Beniro area is outstanding, especially that from the Jerte Valley, where a lot of cherries are grown.

The pastry is typical of a rural cuisine, where flour and lard are used freely. There are *rocas de candelilla, bollos de chicharrones, escaldadillas* (made with dough soaked in orange juice and then fried), *empanadas de bizcocho, bollos de leche,* and *huevillos.*

Estremadura has some good wines, but they are not yet commercialized. They are extremely strong and somewhat wild and are often cloudy with high alcohol content, as well as an unmistakable flavor. The wine from Canamero is only now finding its way into the market. There are also whites from Montánchez, Cillero, Ahigal; and light reds from Hervas.

La Mancha

Like Castile, the cuisine of this area covers many provinces, including Toledo, Albacete, Ciudad Real and, with certain peculiarities of their own, Madrid, Guadalajara and Cuenca. It is a heavy cuisine of long standing.

The cuisine of La Mancha has managed to preserve its character and traditions even today, and to modern tastes it offers very popular and deeply rooted stews and recipes, which is true for most of the famous dishes of Spanish cuisine.

Los gazpachos of La Mancha are a winter dish of huge proportions. Their contents may be traced to the shepherds. They are not found easily in any restaurant along the way, but only in those that are fun and care. Whatever the case, it is not a dish found on the menu at any time of the year.

Like all the others of La Mancha, *los gazpachos* is an ancient recipe mentioned with the name *galianos* in *Don Quixote.* Its time-consuming preparations are almost a rite. First, a large flat piece of unleavened dough must be prepared. It is now sold in Madrid under the name of *torta de Ceceño* from La Roda. The dough is cooked between two sources of heat until it reaches the size of between half a meter and a meter-

and-a-half, depending on the occasion, and remains as thin as the edge of a coin without breaking. Pepper and tomato, rabbit, hare, pigeon, turtledove, chicken or whatever other food at hand is cooked separately. When they are done, small pieces of the dough are added until the gravy is soaked up. The outcome is served on top of an unbroken piece of dough while the meat is put aside and eaten separately. The name *galianos* or *gazpachos* is used exclusively for the pieces of dough soaked in gravy and the shreds of meat from the birds. This is a tasty and very refined dish.

Much more widespread and endlessly imitated is *el pisto manchego*, which has reached national importance and is very much in vogue. There are many varieties, all of Arab origin, but the true *pisto* of La Mancha is made only with red and green peppers, tomatoes and a small amount of squash. Sometimes onion, ham, beaten egg, or marinated tuna are added, but these formulas are capricious.

The cold broth with black olives is called *el moje manchego* which must not be mistaken for *el mojete*, which consists of potatoes sautéed with garlic, paprika, tomato, and bay leaf, to which a poached egg is added.

Other common dishes in typical restaurants of La Mancha include *el asadillo*, roasted red peppers cut in pieces, with a dressing of garlic, tomato and oil; *salpicón*, minced veal with onion, tomato, garlic, parsley and pepper; the popular *ajo arriero* and *el tiznao*, also made with clean shreds of grilled cod, and cooked in a clay dish with pepper, tomato, onion and garlic.

The popular garlic soups with or without cumin and paprika are also made everywhere and will be discussed later. *Las migas de pastor* are not much different from the ones in other places. They are called *canas* if soaked in milk or *mulatas* if soaked in chocolate.

People of La Mancha are very fond of marinated food, meat as well as fish (trout, tuna) or fowl (chicken, partridge). Outstanding is the pickled eggplant which is prepared in

Almagro, following an old Arab formula, and can be found everywhere in central Spain at fairs and taverns.

Then there are some dishes which are exclusive to one province, such as stuffed partridge, *el morteruelo* and *eltojunto*.

Toledo is the province where the red-legged partridge breeds and has become a national and international game species. The bird is stewed using bay leaf, pepper and garlic—and a touch of genius. *El morteruelo* is an impressively solid dish. It is a traditional recipe of the province of Cuenca and is rather rich and tasty with pork liver, giblets, game and a variety of spices. It is reminiscent of pâté because it looks solid and creamy.

Ciudad Real, finally, contributes a very unusual dish to the cuisine of La Mancha. It is called *tojunto*, which is short for *todo junto* ("everything together") and consists of cooking mountain rabbit, garlic, onion, green pepper and a fair amount of olive oil together until everything is done. This dish is found in every province of La Mancha. *El tocrudo* ("everything raw") is similar but presented as a salad. Excellent kid goat is prepared in the province of Guadalajara. It is roasted with thyme and mountain herbs or prepared with garlic.

Madrid

Madrid, although part of La Mancha has a cuisine of its own. It has always had a very complete and reliable range of different cuisines of the whole country, which are magnificently represented. As of late an important series of international cuisines has found its way there as well.

But here we shall stay strictly within the confines of the cuisine of Madrid itself to keep to the purpose of this guide.

The cuisine of Madrid is a combination of the art of cooking of La Mancha and Castile, but adjusted especially to the needs and the character of the capital.

La sopa de ajo or garlic soup is made all over Spain, but it is in Madrid where it has found its place of honor in the cuisine as well as efficient propaganda. The regional versions have not lost a certain air of Madrid in their tasty simplicity. Alexandre Dumas on his visit to Spain was so delighted with this dish that he tried to popularize it in France, where he emphasized its healthy qualities. The truth of the matter is that this soup consists of nothing but bread, garlic, oil and paprika, and all its charm comes from the magic touch of the cook.

Sea bream is a Christmas dish, but it has become popular throughout the year. In Madrid, it is prepared in the oven, sprinkled with bread crumbs and parsley and a few slices of lemon embedded in the fish. It is excellent though it has nothing to do with the ones served in the Basque Country.

The other two Madrid dishes par excellence are chick-pea stew and *callos* (tripe). *Callos a la madrileñas* consist of tripe in a sauce of tomato, onion, bay leaf and thyme. Black pudding, chorizo and small pieces of ham are usually added as well.

And now *el cocido*, the chick-pea stew, which is famous in Madrid and may owe its success to the quality of the famous Lozoya water in which the chick-peas are boiled. It softens the hard chick-pea shell better than any other. It consists of chick-peas, potatoes, cabbage, turnips, beef, marrow bones, streaky bacon, chorizo and black pudding.

On a visit to La Mancha, the different types of cheese fill an important chapter. They are called *manchegos* ("La Mancha cheese") and are made with sheep's milk. They come in two versions: cured and creamy. It is perhaps the most well-known Spanish cheese and can be preserved in a very un-usual fashion: it is put in a receptacle full of oil and in this way the cheese will last up to two years in good condition, apart from acquiring a special and pleasant flavor.

The sausage products of this area are also of good quality.

As for sweets, *mantecados, bollos de aceite* (oily buns) and fried biscuits dipped in honey are plentiful. Especially out-standing are the so-called *bizcocha manchega*, which is a cake soaked in milk, sugar, vanilla, and cinnamon, and *los bizcochos borrachos* (a cake soaked in liqueur). But there is above all the marzipan of Arab origin, made with sugar and almonds.

Regarding wine, La Mancha produces huge quantities of excellent quality. Its *Appellation d'origine* is *Valdepeñas* which one drinks in the course of a *chateo* (which is a mild version of pub-crawling to the tune of a glass of wine or two in each bar) and is supplied to the taverns of Madrid as well as to all the taverns in the area.

Canary Islands

Two products stand out in the agricultural production of the so-called "Fortunate Islands": the tomato and the banana. They are of extraordinary quality, but the cuisine of the Canary Islands is not based on them. It is a cuisine with ancient roots where the influence of the lands of America, present since the discovery, is combined with the cuisine of the Peninsula and of course with the native race of the Guanches, of whom hardly anything is known. Among the oldest recipes handed down from the Guanche past is *el gofio*.

El gofio is a dish which is somewhat reminiscent of the African couscous. It was the staple food of the Canary Islands for a long time. It is made with wheat flour, barley, corn of chick-peas, which are roasted and then mixed with water or milk until a ball of appropriate size is formed. This mixture takes the place of bread with the meal.

The dish reminiscent of the mainland is the stew called *puchero canorio* which is different from the original version because native products are added, among them pumpkin, yam, pear, sweet potato, potato, tender chick-peas.

At times the Canary stew is called *sancocho*, but that is something different. The confusion probably comes from the fact that the term *sancochar* means "to boil." The Canary *sancocho*, however, has nothing to do with the stew. It is made with *sama*, a fresh fish caught in these waters, boiled potatoes and *mojo*.

El mojo is perhaps the most typical recipe of Canary cuisine, because it is found everywhere. It accompanies meat, fish, potatoes and just about anything. It is a dressing made with oil, vinegar, garlic, salt and various spices, depending on the kind of *mojo*: paprika for red *mojo*, piquant peppers for *el mojo picón*, coriander for green *mojo*.

There are a great many broths and soups, especially the popular and original *caldo de jaramago*, which is hedge mustard, and is also used together with watercress in a vegetable stew that is exclusively made in the islands.

Other typical dishes are *el escaldón*, a kind of *pisto*, (mixed vegetables), *las papas arrugas*, which are baked potatoes served with one of the *mojo* varieties. There are also meat loaves and roast chicken with pistachio cream.

One of the sausage products is black pudding prepared as a sweet dish with, believe it or not, sugar, sponge cake and raisins.

In the times of Admiral Drake, the wine of the islands was as famous as sherry and Madeira. Today the different types of wine are acceptable, while the rum is excellent.

The native confectionery is of a very distinct nature: potato, milk and lemon bread, banana cake, yam with honey, *trijaras*, and *turrón de gofio*.

Balearic Islands

The cuisine of the Balearic Islands is no less exotic than that of the Canary Islands. However, this is for other reasons: its ancient roots, its exquisite taste and the imagination that goes into using the ingredients. It is seldom available in public places except if ordered in advance.

There is a clear preponderance of pork and vegetables and a constant inclination towards using a sweet flavor with meats and fish, which is typical of the Mediterranean cuisine.

There is also a sauce which has become internationally famous and which may have been invented on the island— to be more precise, in Menorca, mayonnaise. It must also be pointed out that the cuisine of the three main islands, Majorca, Menorca and Ibiza, has its own characteristics, in each case within a similar framework. Despite the small surface area of these islands, researchers have collected 600 recipes. This is enough to give you an idea of their rich cuisine.

In Majorca, the soups are the most popular. There are two kinds: clear soups, which may be stock from fish, stew, or meat, and the truly Majorcan ones, which are almost solid or dry and are hard to find today. They are probably based on the old cabbage soup and are the best dish in a tame, peaceful rural community of agriculture. They consist of vegetables (mainly cabbage) and slices of bread soaked in stock, apart from paprika, tomato and garlic. The result can be compared to a pudding: light, mild and very juicy.

After the soups, pork comes next. With it an endless number of different dishes is prepared, especially the roasts. It is also prepared with stuffing, which is an incredible mixture of pork liner with eggs, bread, spices, apples and plums. Apart from that, there is the most famous pork product of the islands called *sobrasada*, which has a soft texture and is orange-colored from the paprika.

The best vegetable dish is *el tumbet*, which is a kind of cake with a layer of potato and another of lightly fried eggplant, all of which is covered with tomato sauce and peppers and then boiled for a little while. The eggplant, which is commonly used in this cuisine, is often stuffed with meat or fish and then put in the oven.

Among the recipes with eggs, the dish called *huevos al estilo Soller* is outstanding, The eggs are fried on *sobrasada* and covered with a complicated vegetable-and-milk sauce. And then there is the wonderful stuffed chicken with a pomegranate sauce, breast of turkey with an almond sauce, and turtledove with chestnuts, which are splendid examples of the Majorcan tendency to use sweet flavors with main dishes. As for desserts and pastry, the best is *la ensaimada*, delicate puff pastry which is difficult to make and which is prepared with lard, the same as the numerous and varied crusted pies.

The most important dishes on the island of Menorca are made with fish and seafood, which are plentiful and of great quality along these coasts. *La caldereta de langosta* (a lobster dish) is the most outstanding. It consists of pieces of lobster as well as pepper, onion, tomato, garlic and herb liqueur. Other typical stews on the island are rice with lobster, tuna with mayonnaise, Menorca partridge and baked mutton with *sobrasada*.

In Ibiza the fish dishes predominate as well: *la burrida de ratjada*, boiled skate seasoned with ground almonds; Ibiza lobster with squid and herb liqueur; *el guisat de marisc,* a tasty stew made with a variety of fish and seafood.

And many different types of *coques* are prepared in the Balearics. They are like Catalán pastry (rectangular cakes covered with chopped vegetables, fish of mince meat) and are made all over the Balearic Islands.

Only Majorca produces wine, but other drinks are more interesting in these islands: the gin from Menorca, of English origin, with which the very popular *pellofas* are prepared; and the herb liqueur of Ibiza, which is very strong and should be watered down with ice.

How to Say It:
English to Spanish

Numbers

1	one	uno, una
2	two	dos
3	three	tres
4	four	cuatro
5	five	cinco
6	six	seis
7	seven	siete
8	eight	ocho
9	nine	nueve
10	ten	diez
11	eleven	once
12	twelve	doce
13	thirteen	trece
14	fourteen	catorce
15	fifteen	quince
16	sixteen	dieciséis
17	seventeen	diecisiete
18	eighteen	dieciocho
19	nineteen	diecinueve
20	twenty	veinte
21	twenty-one	veinte y uno
22	twenty-two	veinte y dos
30	thirty	treinta
31	thirty-one	treinta y uno

32	thirty-two	treinta y dos
40	forty	cuarenta
41	forty-one	cuarenta y uno
50	fifty	cincuenta
60	sixty	sesenta
70	seventy	setenta
80	eighty	ochenta
90	ninety	noventa
100	one hundred	cien
101	one hundred one	ciento uno
102	one hundred two	ciento dos
200	two hundred	doscientos, -as
300	three hundred	trescientos, -as
400	four hundred	cuatrocientos, -as
500	five hundred	quinientos, -as
600	six hundred	seiscientos, -as
700	seven hundred	setecientos, -as
800	eight hundred	ochocientos, -as
900	nine hundred	novecientos, -as
1,000	one thousand	mil
2,000	two thousand	dos mil
100,000	one hundred thousand	cien mil
1,000,000	one million	un millón
2,000,000	two million	dos millones

Words and Phrases

AFTER   después
AFTERNOON   tarde
AGAIN   otra vez
ALL RIGHT   De acuerdo
ARE THERE ANY GOOD CHEAP RESTAURANTS AROUND HERE?   ¿Hay algún restaurante bueno y barato cerca de aquí?
ASHTRAY, PLEASE   Páseme el cenicero, por favor
BAKED   al horno

BATHROOM   el baño
BOILED   cocido
BOTTLE   la botella
BREAKFAST   el desayuno
CALL AN AMBULANCE   Llame una ambulancia
CAN YOU HELP ME?   ¿Me puede ayudar?
CAN YOU RECOMMEND A GOOD RESTAURANT?
   ¿Puede recomendar un buen restaurante?
CARAFE   la garrafa
CARRY ON   Continúe
CHANGE   el cambio
CLOSED   cerrado
COLD   frío
CONTINENTAL BREAKFAST   el desayuno continental
COVER CHARGE   el precio del cubierto
CUP   la taza
CUP OF COFFEE   la taza de cafè
DINING ROOM   el comedor
DINNER   la cena, comida
DO YOU SPEAK ENGLISH?   ¿Habla usted inglés?
DO YOU UNDERSTAND?   ¿Comprende usted?
DOES ANYONE SPEAK ENGLISH?   ¿Hay alguien que
   hable inglés?
DON'T MENTION IT   No importa
DRIED   seco
DRINK, TO   beber
DRY   seco
EAT, TO   comer
EMERGENCY   la emergencia
ENTRANCE   la entrada
EXCUSE ME   Discúlpeme
EXIT   la salida
EYEGLASSES   los lentes
FIRE!   ¡Incendio!
FORK   el tenedor
FRIED   frito
GLASS   el vaso

GO MORE SLOWLY   Vaya más lento
GOOD AFTERNOON   Buenas tardes
GOOD DAY   Buenos días
GOOD EVENING   Buenas tardes
GOOD MORNING   Buenos días
GOOD NIGHT   Buenas noches
GOOD-BYE   Adiós
GRILLED   a la parrilla
HEADWAITER   el jefe de meseros
HEART ATTACK   el ataque al corazón
HELLO   Hola
HOSPITAL   el hospital
HOT   caliente
HOTTER   más caliente
HOW   cómo
HOW ARE YOU?   ¿Cómo está usted?
HOW BEAUTIFUL!   ¡Qué bonito es!
HOW MANY?   ¿cuántos?
HUNGRY, TO BE   tener hambre
HURRY UP!   ¡Dese prisa!
I AM WAITING FOR SOMEONE   Estoy esperando a
   alguien
I BEG YOUR PARDON   Perdóneme
I DO NOT KNOW   No lo sé
I HAVE A TOOTHACHE   Me duele el diente
I HAVE LOST MY COAT   Perdí mi abrigo
I LEFT THE TIP ON THE TABLE   Dejé la propina en la
   mesa
I SPEAK ONLY ENGLISH   Hablo inglés solamente
I UNDERSTAND   Yo comprendo
I WOULD LIKE A TAXI   Quiero un taxi
I WOULD LIKE...   Quisiera...
I'M SORRY   Lo siento
I'M VERY SORRY!   ¡Lo siento mucho!
ICE   el hielo
IF YOU PLEASE   Por favor
KEEP THE CHANGE   Quédese con el cambio

KNIFE   el cuchillo
LADIES   las damas
LAVATORY   el lavabo
LIGHT   liviano
LOOK OUT!   ¡Cuidado!
LUNCH   el almuerzo
MARINATED   escabeche
MATCH   fósforo
MEAL   la comida
MEN   los caballeros u hombres
MENU   el menú
MID MORNING SNACK   el refrigerio de media mañana
MISS   señorita
MONEY   el dinero
MORE   más
MR.   señor
MRS.   señora
MY NAME IS...   Me llamo...
NAPKIN   la servilleta
NO   no
PASTRY CART   el carrito de pasteles
PEPPER MILL   el molinillo de pimienta
PHARMACY   la farmacia
PICKLED   escabechado
PIECE   el pedazo
PLATE   el plato
PLEASE   por favor
POACHED   hervido
PREFER, TO   preferir
PRICE   el precio
RARE   poco cocido
RAW   crudo
RESTAURANT   el restaurante
RESTROOMS   los baños
ROASTED   asado
SALTED   salado
SMALL   chico

SMOKED   ahumado
SNACK   el aperitivo
SOUP SPOON   la cuchara sopera
SPOON   la cuchara
STEAMED   cocido al vapor
STEW   el estofado
STOP   Párese
STRAIGHT   sólo
SUPPER   la cena
TABLESPOON   la cuchara grande
TEASPOON   la cucharilla
THANK YOU   gracias
THANK YOU SO MUCH FOR YOUR KINDNESS
    Muchas gracias por su amabilidad
THANK YOU VERY MUCH   Muchas gracias
THIRSTY, TO BE   tener sed
THIS IS WONDERFUL   Esto es maravilloso
TODAY   hoy
TOILET FOR LADIES   el baño de mujeres
TOILET FOR MEN   el baño de hombres
TOMORROW   mañana
TONIGHT   esta noche
TOOTHPICK   el palillo
URGENT   urgente
WAIT FOR ME!   ¡espéreme!
WAITER   camerero *or* mesero
WAITRESS   camerera *or* mesera
WASH, TO   lavar
WATER   el agua
WE ENJOYED IT, THANK YOU   Nos ha gustado, gracias
WE ENJOYED THE MEAL   Nos gustó la comida
WE WOULD LIKE A BOTTLE OF GOOD LOCAL WINE
    Nos gustaría una botella de un buen vino regional
WHERE ARE THE REST ROOMS?   ¿Dónde están los
    baños?
WHO SPEAKS ENGLISH?   ¿Quién habla inglés?
WITHOUT   sin

WRONG   incorrecto, falso
YES   Sí
YOU ARE RIGHT   Usted tiene razón
YOU'RE WELCOME   De nada
YOUR HEALTH!   ¡A su salud!

Food and Drink

A HALF BOTTLE   una media botella
ALMOND   la almendra
ANCHOVY   la anchoa
APERITIF   el aperitivo
APPETIZER   unas tapas, unos saladitos
APPLE   la manzana
APPLESAUCE   el puré de manzana
APRICOT   el albaricoque
ARTICHOKE   la alcachofa
ASPARAGUS   los espárragos
ASSORTED CHEESES   los quesos variados
AVOCADOS   los aguacates
BACON   el tocino
BACON AND EGGS   los huevos con tocino
BAKED IN PARCHMENT   cocido envuelto
BAKED PUFF PASTRY PIE   el pastel
BANANA   el plátano
BEANS   las habichuelas
BEEF   la carne de res
BEEFSTEAK   el bistec
BEER   la cerveza
BEER, BOTTLED   la cerveza embotellada
BEER, DARK   la cerveza oscura
BEER, DRAFT   la cerveza servida directamente del tonel
BEER, LIGHT   la cerveza ligera
BISCUIT   el bizcocho
BLACK COFFEE   el café negro
BLACK OLIVES   las olivas negras
BRANDY   el coñac

BREAD   el pan
BREAKFAST SAUSAGE   la salchicha blanca asturiana
BROAD BEANS   los michirones
BROCCOLI   el brecol *or* bróculi
BURGUNDY   la borgoña
BUTTER   la mantequilla
CABBAGE   el repollo
CAKE   el pastel
CANDY   los dulces
CARP   la carpa
CARROTS   las zanahorias
CAULIFLOWER   la coliflor
CELERY   el apio
CEREAL, COLD   el cereal frío
CEREAL, HOT   el cereal caliente
CHAMPAGNE   el champán
CHEESE   el queso
CHERRIES   las cerezas
CHICKEN   el pollo
CHICKEN FRICASSEE   el fricasé de pollo
CHICKEN, FRIED   el pollo frito
CHICKEN, ROAST   el pollo asado
CHICKEN SOUP   el caldo de pollo
CHIPS (POTATO)   las papitas
CHOCOLATE   el bombón
CHOCOLATE BAR   la barra de chocolate
CHOP   la chuleta
CHOPPED STEAK   el bistec picado
CLAMS   las almejas
COCKTAIL   el cocktail
COD   el bacalao
COFFEE   el café
COFFEE, AMERICAN   el café americano
COFFEE, BLACK   el café solo
COFFEE, DECAFFEINATED   el café descafeinado
COFFEE, ICED   el café helado
COFFEE, INSTANT   el café instantáneo

COFFEE WITH CREAM   el café con crema
COFFEE WITH HOT MILK   el café con leche caliente
COFFEE WITH MILK   el café con leche
COFFEE, ROLLS, BUTTER   el café, los bollos, la mantequilla
COGNAC   el coñac
COLD MILK   la leche fría
CONTINENTAL BREAKFAST   el desayuno continental
COOKIES   las galletas
CORN   el maíz
CRAB   el cangrejo
CRAYFISH   la cigala
CREAM   la crema
CUCUMBER   el pepino
CUSTARD   el flan
DESSERT   el postre
DRY WINE   el vino seco
DUCK   el pato
EEL   el anguila
EGGS   los huevos
EGGS, BOILED   los huevos cocidos
EGGS, BOILED, FIRM   los huevos cocidos firmes
EGGS, BOILED, HARD   los huevos cocidos duros
EGGS, BOILED, SOFT   los huevos tibios
EGGS, FRIED   los huevos fritos
EGGS FRIED OVER   los huevos fritos por dos lados
EGGS FRIED UP   los huevos fritos de un lado
EGGS, FRIED WITH BACON   los huevos fritos con tocino
EGGS, FRIED WITH HAM   los huevos fritos con jamón
EGGS, FRIED WITH POTATOES   los huevos fritos con
    papas
EGGS, FRIED WITH SAUSAGE   los huevos fritos con
    salchichón
EGGS, HARD-BOILED   los huevos duros
EGGS, POACHED   los huevos cocidos al vapor
EGGS, POACHED, FIRM   los huevos escalfados duros
EGGS, POACHED, SOFT   los huevos escalfados suaves
EGGS, SCRAMBLED   los huevos revueltos

EGGS, SCRAMBLED WITH BACON   los huevos revueltos con tocino

EGGS, SCRAMBLED WITH HAM   los huevos revueltos con jamón

EGGS, SCRAMBLED WITH POTATOES   los huevos revueltos con papas

EGGS SCRAMBLED WITH SAUSAGE   los huevos revueltos con salchichón

EGGS WITH BACON   los huevos con tocino

ESPRESSO BLACK   expreso negro

ESPRESSO WEAK   expreso no muy fuerte

ESPRESSO WITH MILK   expreso con leche

FISH   el pescado

FRIED POTATOES   las papas fritas

FROG LEGS   las ancas de rana

FRUIT   la fruta

FRUIT COMPOTE   la compota de fruta

FRUIT DRINK   la bebida de frutas

FRUIT JUICE   el jugo de fruta

FRUIT SALAD   la ensalada de frutas

FULL-BODIED   con mucho cuerpo

GAME   la carne de caza

GARLIC   el ajo

GIN   la ginebra

GIN AND TONIC   la ginebra con tónica

GOOSE   el ganso

GOOSE LIVER PASTE   la pasta de higado de ganso

GRAPE   la uva

GRAPEFRUIT   la toronja

GRAPEFRUIT JUICE   el jugo de toronja

GRAVY   la salsa de carne

GREEN BEANS   las habichuelas verdes

GREEN OLIVES   las olivas verdes

GREEN PEPPER   el pimiento verde

GREEN SALAD   la ensalada verde

GREEN VEGETABLES   los vegetales verdes

HADDOCK   la merluza

HAM   el jamón
HEN   la gallina
HERRING   el arenque
HONEY   la miel
HOT CHOCOLATE   el chocolate caliente
HOT MILK   la leche caliente
HOT WATER   el agua caliente
ICE   el hielo
ICE CREAM   el helado
ICE CUBES   los cubos de hielo
ICE WATER   el agua helada
JAM   la mermelada
JUICE   el jugo
KETCHUP   la salsa de tomate
KIDNEYS   los riñones
LAMB   el cordero
LAMB CHOPS   las chuletas de cordero
LEAN   sin gordo
LEMON   el limón
LEMONADE   la limonada
LETTUCE   la lechuga
LIMA BEANS   los michirones
LIQUEUR   el licor
LIVER   el hígado
LOAF OF BREAD   un pan
LOBSTER   la langosta
MARMALADE, ORANGE   la mermelada de naranja
MASHED POTATOES   el puré de papas
MAYONNAISE   la mayonesa
MEAT   la carne
MEAT OR FISH PIE   las empanadas
MEATBALLS   las albóndigas
MILK   la leche
MINERAL WATER   el agua mineral
MIXED SALAD   la ensalada mixta
MUSHROOMS   los hongos
MUSSELS   los mejillones

MUSTARD   la mostaza
NEAT (STRAIGHT)   derecho
NOODLES   los tallarines
NUT   la nuez
OATMEAL   la avena
OIL   el aceite
OLIVE   la aceituna, el olivo
OLIVE OIL   el aceite de olivo
OMELET   la torta de huevo
ONION   la cebolla
ORANGE   la naranja
ORANGE JUICE   el jugo de naranja
ORANGES   las naranjas
OYSTER   la ostra
PANCAKE   el panqueque
PARSLEY   el perejil
PASTRY   los pasteles
PEACH   el durazno
PEANUTS   los cacahuates
PEAR   la pera
PEAS   los chicharos
PEPPER   el pimiento
PIE   la tarta
PIGEON   el pichón
PIKE   la pica
PINEAPPLE   la piña
PINEAPPLE JUICE   el jugo de piña
PLUM   la ciruela
PORK   la carne de cerdo
PORK CHOPS   las chuletas de cerdo
PORT   oporto
POTATO   la patata
POTATO, BOILED   la papa cocida
POTATOES, FRIED   las patatas fritas
POTATO SALAD   la ensalada de papa
POTATOES, MASHED   el puré de papa
POULTRY   las aves

PRAWNS   los camarones
PRUNES   las ciruelas
RABBIT   el conejo
RADISHES   los rábanos
RASPBERRIES   las frambuesas
RED CABBAGE   la lombarda
RED WINE   el vino tinto
RICE   el arroz
ROAST   el asado
ROAST BEEF   la carne asada
ROAST CHICKEN   el pollo asado
ROAST PORK   el puerco asado
ROAST VEAL   la carne de ternera asada
ROLL   el bollo, el panecillo
ROSÉ WINE   el clarete, el rosado
RUM   el ron
SACCHARIN   la sacarina
SALAD   la ensalada
SALAD DRESSING   el aderezo
SALAMI   el salame, salchichón tipo italiano
SALT   la sal
SALT AND PEPPER   Sal y pimienta
SANDWICH   bocadillo, emparadado, sándwich
SANDWICH ROLLS   los bollos
SAUCE   la salsa
SAUERKRAUT   la col fermentada
SAUSAGE   la salchicha
SAUSAGE LINKS   la salchicha
SCOTCH   el whisky escocés
SCRAMBLED EGGS   los huevos revueltos
SEA BASS   el róbalo
SEAFOOD   los mariscos
SEASONING   los condimentos
SHARK   el tiburón
SHERRY   el jerez
SHRIMP   los camarones
SHRIMP COCKTAIL   el cóctel de camarones

SNAILS   los caracoles
SODA   la soda
SODA WATER   el agua gaseosa
SOFT DRINKS   los refrescos
SOLE   el lenguado
SOUP   la sopa
SPAGHETTI   el espaghetti
SPARKLING   espumoso
SPICY SAUSAGE   la butifarra
SPINACH   las espinacas
SQUID   el calamar
STARTER   las tapas, los saladitos
STEAK   el filete
STEW   el estofado
STRAWBERRIES   las fresas
SUGAR   el azúcar
SWEETS   los dulces
TEA   el té
TEA WITH CREAM   el té con crema
TEA WITH LEMON   el té con limón
TOAST   tostado
TOMATO   el tomate
TOMATO JUICE   el jugo de tomate
TOMATO SAUCE   la salsa de tomate
TONGUE   la lengua
TROUT   la trucha
TRUFFLE   la trufa
TUNA   el atún
TURKEY   el pavo
VANILLA   la vainilla
VEAL   la ternera
VEGETABLE   la legumbre
VEGETABLE SOUP   la sopa de vegetales
VERMOUTH   el vermut
VERY DRY   muy seco
VINEGAR   el vinagre
VODKA   el vodka

WATER   el agua
WATERMELON   la sandía
WHIPPED CREAM   la crema batida
WHISKEY   el whisky
WHISKEY AND SODA   el whisky con soda
WHISKY   el whisky
WHITE WINE   el vino blanco
WINE   el vino
WINE, LOCAL RED   el vino tinto regional
WINE, LOCAL WHITE   el vino blanco regional
WINE, RED   el vino tinto
WINE, SPARKLING   el vino espumante
WINE, VERY DRY   el vino muy seco
WINE, VERY FULL-BODIED   el vino con mucho cuerpo
WINE, WHITE   el vino blanco
YOGURT   el yogurt

In the Restaurant: To Order or Make Requests

A TABLE FOR ..., PLEASE   Una mesa para ..., por favor
A TABLE FOR FOUR, PLEASE   Una mesa para cuatro, por favor
A TABLE FOR THREE, PLEASE   Una mesa para tres, por favor
A TABLE FOR TWO, PLEASE   Una mesa para dos, por favor
AGAIN   otra vez
ANOTHER CHAIR, PLEASE   Otra silla, por favor
ARE THERE ANY GOOD CHEAP RESTAURANTS AROUND HERE?   ¿Hay algún restaurante bueno y barato cerca de aquí?
ARE YOU SERVING BREAKFAST?   ¿Sirven el desayuno?
ARE YOU SERVING DINNER?   ¿Sirven la cena?
ARE YOU SERVING LUNCH?   ¿Sirven la comida?
ARE YOU SERVING TEA?   ¿Sirven el té?
ASHTRAY, PLEASE   Páseme el cenicero, por favor

AT WHAT TIME ARE THE MEALS? ¿A qué hora se sirven las comidas?

BATHROOM el baño

BRING ME THE MENU, PLEASE Tráigame el menú, por favor

BRING ME THE WINE LIST, PLEASE Tráigame la lista de vinos, por favor

BRING US COFFEE NOW Tráiganos el café ahora

CAN I HAVE .... ¿Me puede traer ....

CAN WE DINE NOW? ¿Podemos cenar ya?

CAN YOU HELP ME? ¿Me puede ayudar?

CAN YOU RECOMMEND A GOOD RESTAURANT? ¿Puede recomendar un buen restaurante?

CAN YOU RECOMMEND A GOOD RESTAURANT, NOT TOO EXPENSIVE? ¿Puede recomendar un buen restaurant que no sea muy caro?

CAN YOU TELL ME WHAT THIS IS? ¿Me puede decir qué es esto?

CARAFE OF LOCAL RED WINE, PLEASE Garrafa de vino tinto regional, por favor

CARAFE OF LOCAL WHITE WINE, PLEASE Garrafa de vino blanco regional, por favor

CHAIR la silla

CONTINENTAL BREAKFAST el desayuno continental

COULD I HAVE AN ASHTRAY? ¿Puede darme un cenicero, por favor?

COULD I HAVE ANOTHER CHAIR? ¿Puede darme otra silla, por favor?

COULD WE HAVE A TABLE BY THE WINDOW? ¿Nos puede dar una mesa al lado de la ventana?

COULD WE HAVE A TABLE IN THE CORNER? ¿Nos puede dar una mesa en el rincón?

COULD WE HAVE A TABLE ON THE TERRACE? ¿Nos puede dar una mesa en el patio?

COULD WE HAVE A TABLE OUTSIDE? ¿Nos puede dar una mesa afuera?

COULD WE HAVE A TABLE? ¿Nos puede dar una mesa?

COULD WE HAVE MORE ..., PLEASE?   ¿Nos puede dar
  más ..., por favor?
CUP OF COFFEE   la taza de café
DO YOU ACCEPT TRAVELLER'S CHECKS?   ¿Acepta
  cheques de viajero?
DO YOU HAVE...?   ¿Tienen...?
DO YOU HAVE A CHILDREN'S MENU?   ¿Tienen un
  menú para niños?
DO YOU HAVE A DISH OF THE DAY?   ¿Tiene un plato
  especial del día?
DO YOU HAVE A SET MENU?   ¿Tienen platos combinados?
DO YOU HAVE LOCAL DISHES?   ¿Tienen especialidades
  locales?
DO YOU HAVE SANDWICHES?   ¿Tiene sándwiches?
DO YOU HAVE WINE BY THE GLASS?   ¿Vende vino por
  copa?
FORK   el tenedor
GLASS   el vaso
GLASS OF ..., PLEASE   Un vaso de ..., por favor
GLASS OF BEER   un vaso de cerveza
GLASS OF LIQUEUR   una copa de licor
GLASS OF MILK   un vaso de leche
GLASS OF WATER   un vaso de agua
GLASS OF WINE   una copa de vino
HAVE YOU A TABLE FOR ..., PLEASE?   ¿Tiene una mesa
  para ..., por favor?
HAVE YOU ANY...?   ¿Tiene...?
HAVE YOU COMPLETE DINNERS?   ¿Tiene comida(s)
  completa(s)?
HAVE YOU FIXED PRICE DINNERS?   ¿Tiene comidas
  completas con precio fijo?
HAVE YOU SOMETHING ELSE?   ¿Tiene otra cosa?
HEADWAITER   el jefe de meseros
HOT FIRST COURSES   el primer plato caliente
HOT MAIN COURSES   el plato principal caliente
HOTTER   más caliente
HOW MANY?   ¿cuántos?

HOW MUCH DO I OWE?   ¿Cuánto le debo?

HURRY UP!   ¡Dese prisa!

I AM IN A HURRY   Estoy de prisa

I HAVE HAD ENOUGH, THANKS   Es bastante, gracias

I LIKE THE MEAT MEDIUM   Me gusta la carne medio cocida

I LIKE THE MEAT RARE   Me gusta la carne poco cocida

I LIKE THE MEAT WELL-DONE   Me gusta la carne bien cocida

I WANT   quiero

I WANT A TABLE FOR ... PEOPLE AT ... O'CLOCK
    Quiero una mesa para ... personas a la(s) ...

I WANT SOMETHING SIMPLE, NOT TOO SPICY
    Quiero algo sencillo, no muy condimentado

I WOULD LIKE A BOTTLE OF WINE   Quisiera una botella de vino

I WOULD LIKE A GLASS OF COLD MILK   Quisiera un vaso de leche fria

I WOULD LIKE A GLASS OF RED WINE   Quisiera un vaso de vino tinto

I WOULD LIKE A GLASS OF WHITE WINE   Quisiera un vaso de vino blanco

I WOULD LIKE A GLASS OF WINE   Quisiera un vaso de vino

I'D LIKE A DESSERT, PLEASE   Me gustaría un postre, por favor

I'D LIKE AN APERITIF, PLEASE   Me gustaría un aperitivo, por favor

I'D LIKE AN APPETIZER, PLEASE   Me gustaría un aperitivo, por favor

I'D LIKE SOME BEEF, PLEASE   Me gustaría carne de res, por favor

I'D LIKE SOME FISH, PLEASE   Me gustaría carne de pescado, por favor

I'D LIKE SOME LAMB, PLEASE   Me gustaría carne de cordero, por favor

I'D LIKE SOME PORK, PLEASE   Me gustaría carne de
   puerco, por favor
I'D LIKE TO RESERVE A TABLE FOR ... PEOPLE AT ...
   O'CLOCK   Quiero reservar una mesa para ... a las ...
I'LL TAKE THIS   Tomo esto
INSTEAD   en vez de
IS SERVICE INCLUDED?   ¿Está incluido el servicio?
IS THIS CHEESE MILD OR STRONG?   ¿Este queso es de
   sabor suave o fuerte?
IS THIS RIGHT?   ¿Está bien?
KNIFE   el cuchillo
KOSHER   kosher
LARGE SPOON   la cuchara grande
LEAN   sin gordo
LIGHT   liviano
LOCAL RED WINE   el vino tinto regional
LOCAL WHITE WINE   el vino blanco regional
LOCAL WINE   el vino regional
MATCH   el fósforo
MAY I CHANGE THIS?   ¿Puede cambiarme esto?
MAY I HAVE THIS?   ¿Me trae esto?
MAY I PLEASE HAVE THE MENU?   ¿Puedo ver la carta,
   por favor?
MAY I SPEAK TO...?   ¿Puedo hablar con...?
MAY WE HAVE SOME WATER?   ¿Nos puede traer agua?
MAY WE SIT NEAR THE WINDOW?   ¿Nos podemos
   sentar cerca de la ventana?
MEAL SERVED QUICKLY   la comida servida rápidamente
MEDIUM   el tamaño mediano
MENU   el menú
MID MORNING SNACK   el refrigerio de media mañana
MORE   más
MORE BEER, PLEASE   Más cerveza, por favor
MORE BREAD, PLEASE   Más pan, por favor
MORE COFFEE   más café
MORE, PLEASE   Más, por favor

MORE WATER, PLEASE   Más agua, por favor
NAPKIN   la servilleta
NEED, TO   necesitar
NO SAUCE, PLEASE   Sin aderezo, por favor
NOTHING MORE, THANKS   Es todo, gracias
NOTHING MORE, THANK YOU   Nada más, gracias
ON THE ROCKS   en las rocas
OPEN, TO   abrir
PASTRY CART   el carrito de pasteles
PEPPER MILL   el molinillo de pimienta
PLACE SETTING   poner los lugares individuales en la mesa
PLATE   el plato
PLEASE BRING ME A NAPKIN   Tráigame una servilleta, por favor
PLEASE BRING SOME ICE   Traiga un poco de hielo, por favor
PLEASE HURRY   Por favor, dese prisa
PLEASE SERVE US QUICKLY   Por favor, sírvanos rápido
PLEASE WRITE IT DOWN   Por favor, escríbamelo
POINT TO THE PHRASE IN THIS BOOK   Señale la frase en este libro
PREFER, TO   preferir
PREPARED AT THE TABLE   preparado en su mesa
QUICKLY   rápido, rápidamente
RARE   poco cocido
REQUEST, TO   pedir
SLICE OF   una rebanada de
SMALL   chico
SMALL BOTTLE OF   una botella chica de
SOMETHING LIGHT, PLEASE   Algo ligero, por favor
SOUP SPOON   la cuchara sopera
SPICY SAUCE   el aderezo condimentado
SPOON   la cuchara
TABLE   la mesa
TABLE FOR TWO, PLEASE   Una mesa para dos, por favor
TABLESPOON   la cuchara grande

TAKE IT AWAY, PLEASE   Lléveselo, por favor
TEASPOON   la cucharilla
THAT IS CORRECT   Eso es correcto
THE MENU, PLEASE   La carta, por favor
THE WINE LIST   la lista de vinos
THIRSTY, TO BE   tener sed
TOASTED   tostado
TODAY'S SPECIAL   el plato del día
TOILET FOR LADIES   el baño de mujeres
TOILET FOR MEN   el baño de hombres
TOOTHPICK   el palillo
WAITER   el camarero *or* mesero
WAITRESS   la camarera *or* mesera
WASH, TO   lavar
WE WOULD LIKE A BOTTLE OF DRY WINE   Nos
   gustaría una botella de vino seco
WE WOULD LIKE A BOTTLE OF GOOD LOCAL WINE
   Nos gustaría una botella de un buen vino regional
WE WOULD LIKE A BOTTLE OF RED WINE   Nos
   gustaría una botella de vino tinto
WE WOULD LIKE A BOTTLE OF SWEET WINE   Nos
   gustaría una botella de vino dulce
WE WOULD LIKE A BOTTLE OF WHITE WINE   Nos
   gustaría una botella de vino blanco
WE WOULD LIKE A GLASS OF DRY WINE   Nos
   gustaría una copa de vino seco
WE WOULD LIKE A GLASS OF SWEET WINE   Nos
   gustaría una copa de vino dulce
WELL-DONE   bien hecho *or* bien cocido
WHAT DO YOU RECOMMEND?   ¿Qué recomienda
   usted?
WHAT IS READY NOW?   ¿Qué tiene ya hecho?
WHAT IS THAT?   ¿Qué es eso?
WHAT IS THE LOCAL SPECIALTY?   ¿Cuál es la
   especialidad local?
WHAT IS THE PRICE OF THE MEAL?   ¿Cuánto vale la
   comida?

WHAT IS THE SPECIAL DISH TODAY?   ¿Cuál es el plato
  especial para hoy?
WHAT IS THE SPECIALTY OF THE HOUSE?   ¿Cuál es la
  especialidad de la casa?
WHAT IS THE TIME?   ¿Qué hora es?
WHAT IS THIS?   ¿Qué es esto?
WHAT SALADS DO YOU HAVE?   ¿Qué clase de
  ensaladas tiene?
WHAT SEAFOOD DO YOU HAVE?   ¿Qué clase de
  pescado o mariscos tiene?
WHAT SORTS OF CHEESE HAVE YOU?   ¿Qué clases de
  queso tienen?
WHAT WINE DO YOU RECOMMEND?   ¿Qué vino nos
  recomienda?
WHAT'S THE MATTER?   ¿Qué hay?
WHERE ARE THE REST ROOMS?   ¿Dónde están los baños?
WINE GLASS   el vaso para vino
WINE, VERY FULL-BODIED   el vino con mucho cuerpo
WITH   con
WITH SODA WATER, PLEASE   Con agua de soda, por favor
WITHOUT ICE   sin hielo

Problems

COLD   frío
DIRTY   sucio
FOOD IS COLD   La comida está fría
HARD   duro(a)
HAVE YOU SOMETHING ELSE?   ¿Tiene otra cosa?
HE DOESN'T EAT MEAT   Él no come carne
I AM IN A HURRY   Estoy de prisa
I AM IN A HURRY   Tengo prisa
I AM LOST   Estoy perdido
I ASKED FOR...   He pedido...
I DID NOT ORDER THIS   No pedí esto
I DO NOT LIKE THAT   No me gusta eso
I DO NOT LIKE THIS   No me gusta esto

I DO NOT UNDERSTAND   No comprendo
I HAVE ALREADY PAID   Ya he pagado
I HAVE LOST MY COAT   Perdí mi abrigo
I HAVE LOST MY MONEY   He perdido mi dinero
I HAVE LOST MY PASSPORT!   ¡He perdido mi pasaporte!
I THINK THERE IS A MISTAKE HERE   Creo que hay un
   error aquí
I'M HUNGRY   Tengo hambre
I'M THIRSTY   Tengo sed
IS THERE ANYONE HERE WHO KNOWS FIRST AID?
   ¿Hay alguien aquí que sepa primeros auxilios?
IT DOES NOT TASTE RIGHT   No tiene buen sabor
IT IS NOT GOOD   No está bueno(a)
IT ISN'T HOT ENOUGH   No está suficientemente caliente
MAY I CHANGE THIS?   ¿Puede cambiarme esto?
MEAT IS OVERDONE   La carne está demasiada cocida
MEAT IS TOO RARE   La carne está demasiado cruda
MEAT IS TOUGH   La carne está demasiado dura
MEAT IS UNDERDONE   La carne está media cruda
STOP   Párese
THAT IS BAD   Eso está malo(a)
THAT'S NOT WHAT I ORDERED   Esto no es lo que he
   pedido
THE FISH IS BAD   El pescado está malo descompuesto
THE FOOD IS COLD   La comida está fría
THE MEAT IS BAD   La carne está mala descompuesta
THE MEAT IS OVERDONE   La carne está demasiado
   cocida
THE MEAT IS TOO TOUGH   La carne está dura
THE MEAT IS UNDERDONE   La carne no está bien cocida
THE WINE IS CORKED   El vino está avinagrado
THIS BUTTER IS NOT FRESH   Esta mantequilla no está
   fresca
THIS COFFEE IS COLD   Este café está frío
THIS FORK IS DIRTY   Este tenedor está sucio
THIS IS NOT CLEAN   Esto no está limpio
THIS IS NOT FRESH   Esto no está fresco

THIS IS OVERCOOKED   Esto está muy cocido
THIS IS TOO BITTER   Esto está demasiado amargo
THIS IS TOO SALTY   Esto está demasiado salado
THIS IS TOO SOUR   Esto está muy agrio
THIS IS TOO SWEET   Esto está muy dulce
THIS IS TOO TOUGH   Esto está muy duro
THIS IS UNDERCOOKED   Esto no está bien cocido
THIS MILK IS SOUR   Esta leche está agria
THIS MILK IS WARM   Esta leche está caliente
THIS SPOON IS NOT CLEAN   Esta cuchara no está limpia
THIS TABLECLOTH IS NOT CLEAN   Este mantel no está
   limpio
THIS WINE IS TOO WARM   Este vino está demasiado
   caliente
WOULD YOU ASK THE HEADWAITER TO COME OVER?
   ¿Quiere decirle al jefe de meseros que venga?
WRONG   incorrecto, falso
YOU'VE MADE A MISTAKE IN THIS BILL, I THINK
   Me parece que se ha equivocado en esta cuenta

To Pay

BILL   la cuenta
BILL OR CHECK, PLEASE   La cuenta, por favor
BRING ME THE CHECK, PLEASE   Tráigame la cuenta,
   por favor
CHECK, PLEASE   La cuenta, por favor
COVER CHARGE   el precio del cubierto
DO YOU ACCEPT AMERICAN MONEY?   ¿Acepta dinero
   americano?
DO YOU ACCEPT TRAVELLER'S CHECKS?   ¿Acepta
   cheques de viajero?
DO YOU ACCEPT THE AMERICAN EXPRESS CARD?
   ¿Acepta la tarjeta American Express?
DO YOU ACCEPT DINERS CARDS?   ¿Acepta Diners Cards?
DO YOU ACCEPT MASTER CARD?   ¿Acepta Master Card?
DO YOU ACCEPT VISA CARDS?   ¿Acepta Visa?

HERE IS A TIP   Aquí está una propina
HOW MUCH DO I OWE?   ¿Cuánto le debo?
HOW MUCH IS THAT?   ¿Cuánto cuesta éso?
HOW MUCH MUST I PAY?   ¿Cuánto tengo que pagar?
HOW MUCH?   ¿Cuánto?
I HAVE ALREADY PAID   Ya he pagado
I LEFT THE TIP ON THE TABLE   Dejé la propina en la mesa
I THINK THERE IS A MISTAKE HERE   Creo que hay un
   error aquí
I'D LIKE TO PAY   Quisiera pagar
IS EVERYTHING INCLUDED?   ¿Está todo incluido?
IS SERVICE INCLUDED?   ¿Está incluido el servicio?
IS THIS RIGHT?   ¿Está bien?
KEEP THE CHANGE   Quédese con el cambio
PAY, TO   pagar
PERSONAL CHECKS   los cheques personales
PLEASE CHECK IT   Por favor, compruébelo
PRICE   el precio
SERVICE INCLUDED   El servicio está incluido
SERVICE NOT INCLUDED   El servicio no está incluido
THANK YOU, THIS IS FOR YOU   Gracias, esto es para usted
THAT IS CORRECT   Eso es correcto
THE BILL IS INCORRECT   La cuenta está incorrecta
TIP   la propina
WE ENJOYED THE MEAL   Nos gustó la comida
WE'D LIKE TO PAY SEPARATELY   Quisiéramos pagar
   separadamente
WHAT'S THIS AMOUNT FOR?   ¿A qué corresponde esta
   cantidad?
YOU'RE WELCOME   De nada
YOU'VE MADE A MISTAKE IN THIS BILL, I THINK
   Me parece que se ha equivocado en esta cuenta

Doctor/Dentist/Emergency

CALL A DOCTOR   Llame a un doctor
CALL AN AMBULANCE   Llame una ambulancia

CALL THE POLICE! ¡Llame a la policía!

CAN YOU RECOMMEND A GOOD DENTIST? ¿Puede recomendar a un buen dentista?

DENTIST el dentista

DENTIST, JUST FIX IT TEMPORARILY Arréglelo temporalmente

DOES ANYONE SPEAK ENGLISH? ¿Hay alguien que hable inglés?

EMERGENCY la emergencia

FIRE! ¡Incendio!

HEART ATTACK el ataque al corazón

HELP! ¡Socorro!

HOSPITAL el hospital

I AM ILL Estoy enfermo(a)

I AM LOST Estoy perdido

I HAVE A HEADACHE Tengo dolor de cabeza

I HAVE A STOMACHACHE Tengo dolor de estómago

I HAVE A TOOTHACHE Me duele el diente

IS THERE A DOCTOR HERE? ¿Hay un doctor aquí?

IS THERE ANYONE HERE WHO KNOWS FIRST AID? ¿Hay alguien aquí que sepa primeros auxilios?

IT HURTS HERE Me duele aquí

PHARMACY la farmacia

THERE HAS BEEN AN ACCIDENT Ha sucedido un accidente

THIS IS URGENT Esto es urgente

URGENT urgente

WHEN CAN HE (SHE) COME? ¿Cuándo puede venir?

WHO SPEAKS ENGLISH? ¿Quién habla inglés?

Telephone

CAN I DIAL THIS NUMBER? ¿Puedo marcar este número?

CAN YOU HELP ME GET THE LONG DISTANCE OPERATOR? ¿Me puede ayudar a conseguir la operadora de larga distancia?

DO I NEED TELEPHONE COINS?   ¿Necesito monedas para el teléfono?

EXTENSION NUMBER ..., PLEASE   La extensión ..., por favor

GO MORE SLOWLY   Vaya más lento

HOW MUCH IS A TELEPHONE CALL TO...?   ¿Cuánto cuesta una llamada telefónica a...?

I HAVE BEEN DISCONNECTED   Se desconectó la linea

I WANT TO MAKE A LOCAL CALL TO NUMBER...   Quiero hacer una llamada local al número...

I WANT TO MAKE A PERSON-TO-PERSON CALL TO...   Quiero hacer una llamada de persona a persona a...

I WANT TO MAKE A COLLECT CALL TO...   Quiero hacer una llamada a cobro revertido a...

I WANT NUMBER...   Quiero el numero...

I WOULD LIKE TELEPHONE COINS   Necesito monedas para el teléfono

I WOULD LIKE TO MAKE A LONG-DISTANCE CALL TO...   Quisiera hacer una llamada de larga distancia a...

I WOULD LIKE TO TELEPHONE...   Quisiera telefonear...

MAY I SPEAK TO...?   ¿Puedo hablar con...?

MY NUMBER IS...   Mi número es...

NUMBER IS OCCUPIED   El número está ocupado

OCCUPIED   ocupado

OPERATOR!   ¡Telefonista!

PLEASE ASK HIM (HER) TO CALL ME   Dígale que me llame, por favor

PLEASE CALL A NUMBER   Favor de llamar el número

PLEASE RECONNECT ME   Por favor, me puede conectar otra vez

PLEASE SPEAK MORE SLOWLY   Hable más despacio, por favor

PLEASE TELL HIM (HER) ... CALLED   Por favor, dígale que llamó...

REPEAT, PLEASE   Repita eso, por favor

SPEAKING IS ...   Habla ...

TAXI   el taxi

TELEPHONE   el teléfono
THIS PHONE IS NOT WORKING   No sirve este teléfono
WHAT COIN DO I PUT IN?   ¿Qué moneda uso?
WHAT IS THE TELEPHONE NUMBER?   ¿Cuál es el
   número telefónico?
WHERE IS THE TELEPHONE BOOK?   ¿Dónde está la
   guía telefónica?
WHERE IS THERE A TELEPHONE?   ¿Dónde hay un
   teléfono?

3

How to Understand It: Spanish to English

Appetizers

ACEITUNAS NEGRAS   black olives
ACEITUNAS VERDES   green olives
AGUACATE RELLENO DE GAMBAS CON ADEREZO
   avocado filled with prawns in a mayonnaise sauce
ALBÓNDIGAS   pork meatballs
ALBÓNDIGAS MAYONESA   pork meatballs with
   mayonnaise garlic dip
ALIÑADAS NEGRAS   black olives
ALIÑADAS VERDES   green olives
ALMEJAS   clams
ALMEJAS AL HORNO   baked stuffed clams
ALMEJAS ENDIABLADAS   clams in a spicy tomato sauce
ALMEJAS MARINERAS   clams in hot pimento sauce
ALMEJAS ROMESCO   clams in tomato sauce with hot
   pepper, chili pepper, vinegar and garlic
ALVERJINES FARCIDES ANXOVE   stuffed eggplant with
   anchovy
ANCAS DE RANA   frog's legs
ANCAS DE RANA A LA PROVENZAL   frog's legs
   sauteed in olive oil, garlic and parsley
ANCHOVAS FRITAS   deep fried anchovies
ANGUILA AHUMADA   smoked eel
ARENQUE   herring
ARENQUE AHUMADO   kippered herring

ARENQUE ESCABECHE   pickled herring
ATÚN ESCABECHADO   pickled tuna fish
AVE   bird
BANDERILLAS   toothpicks with bits of delicacies, such as
    pickled vegetables, ham, cheese, smoked fish
BARCOS DE ANCHOAS   anchovy boat tarts
BOLETA GRAELLA   grilled wild mushroom
BOQUERONES   smelts fish like a large anchovy
BOQUERONES EN VINAGRE   smelts marinated in garlic
    vinegar
BOQUERONES EN VINAGRE FRITOS   fish marinated in
    garlic vinegar and fried
BRANDADA BACALLA   salt cod puree
BRANDADA CARXOFE   salt cod puree with artichoke
BUÑUELITOS CHORIZO   fritters made with chopped
    sausage
BUÑUELITOS DE BACALAO   cod fritters
BUÑUELITOS DE HUEVO DURO   hard-boiled egg fritters
BUÑUELITOS DE JAMÓN   ham fritters
BUÑUELITOS DE POLLO   chicken fritters
BUNYOL DE BACALLA   salt cod fritter
BUNYOL DE CIURENY   wild mushroom fritter
CALAMARES   squid
CALAMARES RELLENOS   squid fried in oil and stuffed
    with chopped ham
CALAMARES ROMANOS   squid slices fried in batter
CALAMARES SALTEJATS ALL JULIVERT   squid sauteed
    with garlic
CALAMARES TINTOS   squid braised in its own ink
CALCOT FRITAS   deep fried green onion
CANAPE   toasted or fried crustless bread covered with a
    spread
CARACOL   snail
CARGOLADA   grilled snails
CEBOLLITAS RELLENAS   small stuffed onions
CHAMPIÑONES AJILLO   mushrooms stir-fried in olive
    oil with garlic chili pepper

CHAMPIÑONES JEREZ, EN   mushrooms sauteed in
    sherry wine
CHAMPIÑONES RELLENOS   pork stuffed baked
    mushrooms
CHAMPIÑONES SALTEADOS   mushrooms sauteed in
    garlic butter
CHAMPIÑONES SEGOVIANA   mushrooms sauteed in
    wine, garlic and bacon
CHORIZO CON SIDRA   sausage and apples in hard cider
    sauce
CHORIZO HOJALDRADO   sausage slices baked in pastry
COCA DE ANEE OLIVES   duck and olive pastry
CÓCTEL DE CAMARONES   shrimp cocktail
CÓCTEL DE GAMBAS   prawn cocktail
CÓCTEL DE MARISCOS   cocktail of various seafoods
CONCHAS FINAS   medium size clams
CONGRI MUSSOLINA ALL   chick-peas with garlic
    hollandaise sauce
COQUINAS   small clams
COTZE   mussel
CROQUETAS GAMBAS, DE   fried balls of shrimp
    croquettes
CROQUETAS PAELLA, EN   fried balls of paella rice
    mixture
EMPANADILLAS DE CHORIZO   chorizo sausage pastries
EMPANADILLAS JAMÓN   ham pastries
EMPANIDILLAS VALENCIANAS   pastries stuffed with
    ham and tuna
ENSALADA ARENQUE, DE   herring salad
ENSALADA COLAS DE CANGREJO, DE   crayfish salad
ENTRADAS   light appetizers
ENTRANTES   appetizers
ENTREMESES   hors-d'oeuvres, first courses
ENTREMESES CORRIENTES   appetizers of seasonal local
    ingredients
ENTREMESES DE MAR   seafood appetizers
ENTREMESES DEL MESÓN   appetizers of the restaurant

ENTREMESES DEL PUERTO   seafood appetizers
ENTREMESES ESPECIALES   restaurant specialties
ENTREMESES SURTIDOS   assorted appetizers
ENTREMESES VARIADOS   assorted cold appetizers
ESCABECHE   pickled
ESCABECHE SARDINES   pickled sardines
ESPÁRRAGOS DOS SALSAS, CON   asparagus with two
   sauces
ESTURIÓN   sturgeon
FARCELLETS COL   pork and cabbage dumplings
FLAMENQUINES   pork and ham slices fried and served
   in white sauce
FLAN ALBERGINIES, DE   eggplant flan
FLAN PEUADA, DE   pigs' feet mousse
FOIE GRAS FRANCÉS   French goose liver pate
FRITOS   fried appetizers
GAMBAS AJILLOS, CON   shrimp with garlic mayonnaise
   sauce
GAMBAS, CÓCTEL DE   shrimp cocktail with mayonnaise
   sauce
GAMBAS GARBARDINA, CON   fried shrimp in a beer
   batter coating
GAMBAS MAYONESA, CON   shrimp cocktail
GAMBAS SALSA PIPARRADA, CON   shrimp with
   tomato and pepper sauce
GAMBAS VILLEROY   boiled shrimp in a white bechamel
   sauce
GAROM   anchovy-olive pâté
GELATINA AVE   cold, poached chicken stuffed with
   meat, rolled, covered with gelatin
GUACAMOLE   pureed avocado, onion and seasonings
HIGADILLOS GELE OPORTO   chicken livers in port
   flavored aspic
HUEVAS ALIÑADAS   seasoned fish roe
HUEVOS MAYONESA   hard-boiled eggs with mayonnaise
HUEVOS RELLENOS CON SALMÓN   salmon stuffed
   hard eggs

JAMÓN AÑEJO CON PEPINILLOS   aged ham with pickles
JAMÓN CANUTILLOS, CON   slices of ham rolled and
   filled
JAMÓN DULCE   ham boiled and served cold
JAMÓN, LONCHAS DE   thin slices of ham
JAMÓN MELÓN, Y   ham and melon
JAMÓN TACOS, EN   diced ham
JAMÓN VARIANTE   sliced ham with various garnishes
JAMÓN VIRUTAS   thin slices of ham
LANGOSTINOS CLAVO, CON   boiled large shrimp in
   wine, pepper, clove, peppercorn sauce
MEJILLONES   mussels marinated in oil, vinegar, capers,
   onion
MEJILLONES CON SALSA VERDE   mussels in wine, oil,
   onion, garlic sauce
MEJILLONES GRATINADOS   baked mussels and
   mushrooms
MELÓN JAMÓN, CON   melon with raw cured ham
MELÓN OPORTO   melon flavored with port wine
MOUSSE FETGE POLLASTRE   chicken liver mousse
MUSCO GRATINATS   gratineed mussel
OSTRAS   oysters
OSTRAS, 1/2 DOCENA DE   half a dozen oysters
PA TOMAQUET   tomato bread
PALITOS   toothpicks with bits of delicacies, such as
   pickled vegetables, ham, cheese, smoked fish
PAMBOLI TOMATIGA   tomato bread
PASTA DE HÍGADO DE GANSO   goose liver pâté
PASTA HOJALDRADA   filled puff pastry
PASTELILLO   little tart
PATATE CATALANA   stuffed potato
PATATE RABASSOLE   potato with mushroom
PATÉ CAMPO, DE   country-style pâté
PATÉ CASOLANA   home style pâté
PATÉ FOIE GRAS   goose liver pâté
PEBRE FARCITS ANEC   sweet red pepper stuffed with
   duck

PEBRE FARCITS PORC I CALAMARS   sweet red pepper
  stuffed with pork and squid
PEBRE PIQUILLO FARCITS CON BRANDADA BACALLA
  sweet red pepper stuffed with salt cod puree
PERCEBES   goose barnacles
PESC VI I SALVIA   fish with wine and sage
PESCADITOS CON ESCABECHE A LA CATALANA
  fried small marinated fish with pepper and garlic
PESCADITOS CON ESCABECHE A LA ANDALUZA
  fried small marinated fish Andalusian style, with saf-
  fron, ginger and garlic
PETITS FULLATS COTLLIURE   anchovy butter canapés
PETITS PASTISOS SAMFAINA ANXOVES   mixed vege-
  table tarts with anchovies
PINCHO   broiled meat or mushrooms cooked on a skewer
PINCHO MORUNO   seasoned pork cubes grilled on a
  skewer
PIOS NONOS   chicken and potato croquettes
POMES FARCIDES   pork stuffed apples
PULPO   octopus
PULPO GALLEGO   octopus boiled in a sauce of paprika,
  pepper, garlic, olive oil
PULPO VINAGRETA, A LA   octopus boiled and mari-
  nated in wine vinegar, served cold
RAVAS   bits of fried octopus
REGAÑAOS   pastry with sardines and red pepper in the crust
SALCHICHA RELLENA CON REPOLLO   sausage fried
  in cabbage leaf
SALMÓN AHUMADO   smoked salmon
SARDINAS ACEITE   sardines canned in oil
SEVICHE   raw fish with onions, garlic
TAPAS CABRALE Y PIÑONES   blue cheese and pine nut
  spread on toast
TAPAS DE ANCHOA Y PIMIENTO   anchovy and
  pimento spread on toast
TARTALETAS   pastry crust filled with cream sauce
  mixture of seafood, chicken or meat

TARTALETAS CON CHAMPIÑÓN   pastry tarts filled with mushrooms

TARTALETAS CON SALMÓN   pastry tarts filled with salmon

TARTINA   slice of buttered bread topped with a filling

TESTÍCULOS TORO ALLI I JULIVERT   bull testicles with garlic and parsley

TORTILLITAS CON CAMARONES   shrimp pancakes

VIVAS   raw oysters on the half shell

Beverages

AGUA   water

AGUA GASEOSA   soda water

AGUA MINERAL   mineral water

AGUA NATURAL   plain water

ANDALUCÍA   dry sherry and orange juice

ANISADO   slightly alcoholic aniseed based soft drink

BATIDO   milk shake

BEBIDA   drink

CACAO   cocoa

CAFÉ   coffee

CAFÉ CORTADO   strong coffee in a small cup with dash of milk

CAFÉ DESCAFEINADO   decaffeinated coffee

CAFÉ EXPRES   espresso, small cup of strong black coffee

CAFÉ GRANIZADO   iced coffee with milk

CAFÉ CON LECHE   coffee with milk

CAFÉ NEGRO   black coffee

CAFÉ SIN LECHE   coffee without milk

CAFÉ SOLO   black coffee

CHOCOLATE   hot milk and chocolate, boiled and whipped

CHOCOLATE CON LECHE   hot chocolate with milk

COLA DE MONO   coffee, milk, rum and grape brandy

CREMA   cream

CREMAT   liqueur laced cinnamon coffee with heavy cream

GARRAFA   carafe
GASEOSA   carbonated water
HIELO   ice
HORCHATA   almond or coconut flavored soft drink
   served cold
HORCHATA DE ALMENDRA   drink made of ground
   almonds
JUGO   juice
JUGO NARANJA, DE   orange juice
JUGO PIÑA, DE   pineapple juice
JUGO TOMATE, DE   tomato juice
JUGO TORONJA, DE   grapefruit juice
LECHE   milk
LIMONADA   lemonade
LIMONADA MADRILEÑA   red wine, lemon juice, peach
   and lemon wedges and water
MAZAGRÁN   lemon flavored iced coffee
MOKA   mocha coffee
NARANJADA   orangeade
NATA   cream
NO-ALCOHÓLICO   non-alcoholic
PONCHE CON COÑAC   hot milk, almond and brandy
   drink
REFRESCO   soft drink
SANGRÍA   drink of red wine, orange liqueur and fresh
   fruit pieces
SANGRÍA BLANCA   drink of white wine, orange liqueur
   and fresh fruit pieces
SELTZ   soda water
SIDRA   cider
SORBETE   iced fruit drink
TAZA DE CAFÉ   cup of coffee
TÉ   tea
VASO   glass
VASO DE AGUA   glass of water
VASO DE LECHE   glass of milk
YERBA MATE   South American holly tea

ZUMO   juice
ZUMO FRUTA   fruit juice
ZUMO LIMÓN   lemon juice
ZUMO NARANJA   orange juice
ZUMO POMELO   grapefruit juice

Breads

BOCADILLO   sandwich
BOLLITO   roll
BOLLO   roll or cake
BROA   Portuguese cornbread
CHURRO MADRILEÑO   crisp fried cruller
COQUE   pizza
EMPAREDADO   sandwich
EMPAREDADO CALIENTE   hot sandwich like French
   toast with ham filling
GALLETA   biscuit *or* cracker
GOFIO   wheat flour, barley, corn or chick-peas, mixed
   with milk until a ball is formed
LA ROSTA   thick bread slices toasted with garlic spread
   then dipped in hot olive oil
MANTECADAS ASTORGA   cinnamon muffins
MASSA SOBADA   Portuguese sweet bread
MEDIAS NOCHES   small buns often used for tea sand-
   wiches or snacks
MIGAS   bread soaked in water, fried with bacon and dry
   peppers
PA TOMAQUET   tomato bread
PAMBOLI TOMATIGA   tomato bread
PAN   bread
PAN CANDEAL   country style bread, slightly sour
PAN CEBADO   strong flavored corn and barley bread
PAN GALLEGO DE CENTENO   round rye bread
PAN PUEBLO, DE   white bread loaf
PAN QUEMADO   sweet bread with baked egg white
   topping

PAN SANTA TERESA   French toast
PAN TOSTADO   toasted bread
PANECILLO   French roll
PICATOSTE   deep fried bread
SUIZO   bun
SUIZOS   baked sugar topped breakfast sweet rolls
TARTINA   slice of buttered bread topped with a filling
TORRIJAS   French toast
TORRIJAS CON VINO   wine-dipped French toast
TORTA CHICHARRONES, CON   baked bread with
   crunchy pork fat pieces, sugar, egg and lemon rind
TORTELES   baked, almond paste filled, sweet bread rings
TOSTADA   toast
TOSTADO   toast

Cakes and Pastries

ALFAJORES   filled cookie dessert
ALMENDRADOS   almond cookies
BARQUILLOS   round cookie pastries
BARTOLILLOS   custard filled fried pastry made with
   wine, lemon peel, cinnamon
BIZCOCHITOS   crackers, cookies
BIZCOCHUELO   cake
BIZCOCHA MANCHEGA   cake soaked in milk, sugar,
   vanilla and cinnamon
BIZCOCHO   cake
BIZCOCHO ALMENDRAS   almond sponge cake
BIZCOCHO BORRACHO   sponge cake with rum, wine or
   syrup
BIZCOCHO BORRACHO CREMA   liqueur flavored cake
   with custard filling
BIZCOCHO CREMA   sponge cake with cream filling
BIZCOCHO GENOVESO   ladyfingers
BIZCOCHOS   sweet biscuits
BIZCOCHOS BORRACHOS   tea cakes with caramelized
   sugar and wine

BIZCOTELA   glazed cookie
BOLO DE ALMENDRA ALGARVIA   almond layer cake
BOLO REY   candied fruit and nut bread
BRAZO GITANO   sponge cake roll with rum cream filling
BREVAS SORIA   custard filled small doughnuts
BUÑUELO   fritter *or* doughnut
BUÑUELOS   sweet fritters; also see BUNYOL and BUÑUELO
BUÑUELOS CON LIMÓN   lemon crullers
BUNYOL   fried pastry
CANAS   fried pastry cylinders filled with cream or custard
CASADIELLES   baked puff pastry horns filled with walnut mixture
CHURRO   deep-fried doughnut
CHURRO MADRILEÑO   crisp fried cruller
ENSAIMADA   baked, sugar topped, snail shaped sweet rolls
FAYULES   flat cakes
FLAO   mint and cream cheese tart
FLAON   honey cheesecake with anisette liqueur and mint
GALLETA   biscuit *or* cracker
GALLETA CON NATA   sandwich cookie with cream center
GATO FORMATGE   cheesecake
GRANADINAS   baked almond cinnamon cookies
HOJALDRA   puff pastry used for dessert or with fillings of meat and fish
LENGUAS DE GATO   wafer thin crisp cookies served with ice cream or custard
LLAMINADURE   pastry, dessert, sweet
MANTECADAS ASTORGA   cinnamon muffins
MANTECADOS   cookies
MASITAS   cupcakes
MASSA SOBADA   Portuguese sweet bread
MIL HOJAS CREMA   pastry layered with custard and frosted on top
MOSTACHONES   small cakes for dipping in coffee or hot chocolate
NEULE   rolled cookie
OVAS MOLES   egg yolk icing

PAN MUNICIÓN   chocolate custard cake with chocolate
    sauce
PANELLET   marzipan cookie
PANELLETS   Catalán almond cookies
PASTAS   pastry
PASTEL HOJALDRADO   puff pastry *or* cream puff
PASTEL NUECES, CON   puff pastry with chopped nuts
PASTEL SUIZO   individual pastries sprinkled with sugar
PASTEL YEMA HELADO   pastry made with egg yolk and
    sugar cream filling, frozen
PASTELERÍA   pastry *or* pastry shop
PASTELERÍA FINA   delicate pastry
PASTELES   cakes
PASTELES FRUTAS, DE   fruit tarts
PASTELES HIGOS, CON   baked puff pastry with fig and
    candied squash filling
PASTELILLO   little tart
PASTELITOS   small cakes
PESTIÑOS   honey covered fritter
PESTIÑOS ANDALUCES   crullers with lemon and anise
    liqueur
PETITSOUS   chocolate eclair
POLVORÓN   hazelnut cookie
POLVORONES   cinnamon cookies
POLVORONES SEVILLANOS   brandy flavored butter
    cookies
PONCHE SEGOVIANO   spongecake soaked in liquor
    with cream filling
QUEIJADAS EVORA   sweet cheese tarts
QUESADA   sweet made with fresh cheese, honey and
    butter
RELÁMPAGOS   pastry-like eclair, with filling
ROSCAS   a cookie
ROSQUILLA   doughnut
ROSQUILLAS RÍO JANAS   small doughnuts made with
    wine, anise and sugar
RUSOS   cake with custard filling cut in squares

SOBADOS PASIEGOS   pastry rich in butter and eggs
SUIZO   bun
TARTA ALMENDRAS, DE   almond cake
TARTA CAPUCHINA   spongecake with custard topping
TARTA CONVENTO, DE   puff pastry tart with chocolate
   glaze
TARTA GALLEGA   almond cake
TARTA HUERTO CURA, DEL   cake with frozen orange
   custard and orange liqueur
TARTA MANTEQUILLA, DE   cookies *or* spongecake
   spread with a chocolate butter cream filling, meringue,
   nuts and fruits
TARTA MANZANA, DE   open face apple cake with
   custard inside
TARTA MIL HOJAS   Napoleon
TARTA NARANJA, CON   orange almond cake with
   orange syrup
TARTA NORMANDA   cake made with apples
TARTA NUECES, CON   chocolate cake with chopped nuts
TARTA PIÑONES, CON   tart with pine nuts
TARTA PONCHE, CON   layered cake with cream filling
   and chopped almonds
TARTA QUESO, DE   cheesecake
TARTA SANTIAGO   almond cake with almond topping
TARTA YEMAS, CON   cake with liquor soaked sponge cake
TECLA CON YEMA   baked puff pastry horns with
   candied egg yolk filling
TOCINILLO CIELLO   sweet made with egg yolk and sugar
TORTA MOCA, DE   mocha layer cake with rum
TORTAS ACEITE, CON   anise and sesame seed cookies
TORTERA   pastry
TOUCINHO CEU   almond cake

Cheese

AJOQUESO   melted cheese, peppers, etc.
ASTURIAS   strong, sharp cheese

BURGOS   soft, creamy cheese
CABRALES   blue cheese
CAMEMBERT CON JITOMATE CONFITURA   fried
  camembert with tomato preserves
CEBRERO   blue-veined, creamy, sharp cheese
CINCHO   hard cheese
MANCHEGO   Spanish cheese
PARMESANA   Parmesan cheese
PERILLA   bland cheese
QUESO   cheese
QUESO BANDEJA, EN   tray of assorted cheese
QUESO DEL PAÍS   cheese of the area
QUESO ELEGIR   cheese of your choice
QUESO EXTRANJERO   imported cheese
QUESO GALLEGO   medium-soft cheese
QUESO NATA, DE   cream cheese
QUESO, PLATO DE   plate of cheese
QUESO, TABLA DE   a cheese board
QUESOS SURTIDOS   assorted cheeses
REQUESÓN   soft, white cheese
REQUESÓN CON MIEL   cottage cheese with honey
RONCAL   spicy hard cheese made from sheep's milk
SAN SIMÓN   firm bland cheese
TABLA   cheese board
ULLOA   soft cheese like camembert
VILLALÓN   cheese from sheep's milk

Desserts, Fruits, and Nuts

AGUACATE   avocado
ALASKA LLAMAS   flamed Baked Alaska
ALBARICOQUE   apricot
ALFAJORES   filled cookie dessert
ALMENDRA   almond
ALMENDRA GARRAPINADA   sugared almond
ALMENDRADOS   almond cookies
ALMENDRAS GARRAPIÑADAS   honey glazed almonds

ALMÍBAR   syrup

ALVERJINES DULCES   fried eggplant with honey

AMETLLE   almond

ANACARDIOS   cashew nuts

ARLEQUÍN DE FRESA Y VAINILLA   ice cream of strawberry and vanilla

ARROZ DOCE   rice pudding

ARROZ LECHE ASTURIANO, CON   rice pudding with
anisette, cinnamon, boiled down milk, brandy

ARROZ LECHE GALLEGO, CON   rice pudding with
caramelized coating

ARROZ LECHE, CON   rice pudding

AVELLANA   hazelnut

AZUCADA   sprinkled with sugar

BABARRÚA CON NARANJA MORA   frozen orange
custard with blackberry sauce

BANDA CON ALMENDRAS   almond and marmalade
puff pastry

BANDEJA   tray

BARQUILLOS   round cookie pastries

BISCUIT CON NUECES Y SALSA DE FRAMBUESA   ice
cream dessert with chopped walnuts and raspberry
sauce

BISCUIT GLACE   ice cream dessert

BISCUITS   molded frozen desserts

BIZCOCHITOS   crackers, cookies

BIZCOCHUELO   cake

BIZCOCHA MANCHEGA   cake soaked in milk, sugar,
vanilla and cinnamon

BIZCOCHO ALMENDRAS   almond spongecake

BIZCOCHO BORRACHO   spongecake with rum, wine or
syrup

BIZCOCHO BORRACHO CREMA   liqueur flavored cake
with custard filling

BIZCOCHO CREMA   spongecake with cream filling

BIZCOCHO GENOVESO   ladyfingers

BIZCOCHOS   sweet biscuits

BIZCOCHOS BORRACHOS   tea cakes with caramelized sugar and wine

BIZCOTELA   glazed cookie

BLANCO NEGRO   chocolate pudding covered with whipped cream

BOCADILLOS DE MONJA   almond and egg yolk candies

BOLO DE ALMENDRA ALGARVIA   almond layer cake

BOLO REY   candied fruit and nut bread

BOMBA   molded frozen dessert

BOMBA MERCEDES   mold with apricot ice and a custard mixture with Chartreuse liquor

BOMBÓN   chocolate

BOMBONES HIGOS   fig candies with almonds

BORRACHUELOS   fried pastry with licorice flavor and sesame seeds

BRAZO GITANO   spongecake roll with rum cream filling

BREVAS   black figs

BUDÍN   pudding

BUÑUELO   fritter *or* doughnut

BUÑUELO CON CREMA   fried doughnut, filled with cream or custard

BUÑUELOS CON LIMÓN   lemon crullers

BUÑUELOS CON MANZANA   apple fritters

BUÑUELOS CON PLÁTANO   deep fried banana fritters

BUNYOL   fried pastry

CABELLOS DE ÁNGEL CALABACÍN   made of pumpkin squash, cooked in flavored sugar syrup

CACAHUETE   peanut

CAMEMBERT CON JITOMATE CONFITURA   fried camembert with tomato preserves

CANAS   fried pastry cylinders filled with cream or custard

CANASTILLA DE FRUTA   small basket of fruit

CANASTILLA FRUTAS   basket of fresh fruit

CANUTILLOS   baked puff pastry horns filled with custard

CAPIROTADA   sweet bread pudding with cinnamon

CAQUI   persimmon

CARAMELO   caramel

CARNE MEMBRILLO, DE   sweet fruit paste

CARRO   food cart

CASADIELLES   baked puff pastry horns filled with walnut mixture

CASATA NAPOLITANA   molded ice cream, with strawberry and praline ice cream, crumbled macaroons, candied fruit, maraschino liqueur

CASTAÑA   chestnut

CEREZA   cherry

CESTA DE FRUTA   basket of fresh fruit

CESTA FRUTAS   basket of fresh fruit

CHABACANO   apricot

CHUMBO   prickly pear

CIRUELA   plum

CIRUELA PASA   prune

CLAUDIA   greengage plum

COCO   coconut

CÓCTEL DE FRUTA   fruit cocktail

COMPOTA   stewed fruit

COMPOTAS   fruits preserved in syrup

CONFITURA   jam

COPA ALEJANDRA   mixed fruits in kirsch liquor with strawberry ice cream and strawberries

COPA AMERICANA   pineapple ice with crushed pineapple and macaroons, covered with whipped cream and crystallized fruits

COPA MELBA   poached peach and vanilla ice cream, covered with raspberry sauce and whipped cream

COPA NURIA   whipped eggs served with jam

COPA PEÑASANTA   Baked Alaska for one

COPA VENUS   vanilla ice cream with poached peach, strawberry and whipped cream

COPAS   ice cream sundaes

CREMA BATIDA   whipped cream

CREMA CATALANA   cream custard with cinnamon or candied sugar coating

CREMA CATALANA CON CARAMELO   baked custard
  with burned caramel crust
CREMA DAMA BLANCA   vanilla ice cream
CREMA DAMA DIABLO TÚNICA   vanilla ice cream
  with chocolate sauce
CREMA DAMA PURPÚREO   vanilla ice cream with
  strawberry sauce
CREMA ESPAÑOLA   gelatin and egg dessert
CREMA INGLESA   frothy cooked custard
CREMA JEREZ, DE   chocolate sherry chiffon pudding
CREMA NARANJA, DE   orange cream custard
CREMA NIEVE, DE   beaten egg yolk, sugar and rum
CREMA PASTELERA RON   rum cream filling
CREMA QUEMADA   caramelized custard filling
CREPES CREMA   custard filled pancakes
CREPES SUZETTE   spread with filling flavored with
  orange juice, Cointreau, flamed with cognac
CROCANTI   chopped almonds in caramel
CUAJADA LECHE   junket of ewe's milk
CUAJADA MIEL   rennet pudding with honey and walnuts
DAMASCO   kind of apricot
DÁTIL   date
DULCE DE MEMBRILLO   quince marmalade
DURAZNO   peach
ENSAIMADA   baked, sugar topped, snail shaped sweet
  rolls
ESPUMA CHOCOLATE   frothy chocolate pudding
FATIAS CHINAS   egg and almond slices in syrup
FIGOS RECHEADOS   dried figs stuffed with almonds
  and chocolate
FIGUES   figs
FILLOAS CON CREMA   thin dessert pancake filled with
  custard
FLAN   dessert of egg custard with caramel sauce
FLAN CARAMELO, CON   caramelized baked custard
FLAN CASERO   homemade custard
FLAN COCO, DE   caramelized coconut custard

FLAN CREMOSO   boiled custard
FLAN DOBLE   double portion of flan
FLAN GRAN FLANERO   caramel custard
FLAN HUEVO, DE   egg custard
FLAN MANZANA CON PURÉ DE FRESA, DE   apple
   flan with strawberry puree
FLAN NARANJA, DE   orange caramel custard
FLAN UNIDAD   individual molded custard
FLAO   mint and cream cheese tart
FLAON   honey cheese cake with anisette liqueur and mint
FRAMBUESA   raspberry
FRAMBUESA NATA   raspberry with cream
FRAMBUESA SILVESTRE   wild raspberry
FRESA   strawberry
FRESA BORRACHA   strawberry with liquor
FRESA BOSQUE   wild strawberry
FRESA CON NATA   strawberry with cream
FRESA SILVESTRE   wild strawberry
FRESÓN   large strawberry
FRUTA   fruit
FRUTA ESCARCHADA   candied fruit
FRUTA MIXTA   assorted fruits
FRUTA SARTÉN, DE   dessert fritter
FRUTA SECA   dried fruit
FRUTA TIEMPO   fruit in season
GALLETA CON NATA   sandwich cookie with cream center
GATO FORMATGE   cheesecake
GELATINA CANYELLA   cinnamon ice cream with
   strawberry
GRANADA   pomegranate
GRANADINAS   baked almond cinnamon cookies
GRANIZADO   shaved ice over strong, sweetened coffee
   or fruit syrup
GRENADILLA   passion fruit
GROSELLA   currant
GROSELLA ESPINOSA   gooseberry
GROSELLA NEGRA   black currant

GROSELLA ROJA   red currant

GUAYABA   guava

GUINDA   sour cherry

HELADO   ice cream *or* any frozen dish

HELADO CHOCOLATE, DE   chocolate ice cream

HELADO CIRUELA PASA, DE   prune ice cream in orange
  liqueur sauce

HELADO HORNO, AL   Baked Alaska

HELADO JIJONA, CON   vanilla ice cream mixed with
  nougat candy

HELADO NATA, CON   ice cream with whipped cream

HELADO SEMIFRÍO   molded frozen dessert

HELADO TURRÓN, DE   vanilla ice cream with nougat
  candy mixed in

HELADO VAINILLA, DE   vanilla ice cream

HELADOS VARIADOS   various flavors of ice cream

HIGO   fig

HUEVAS NIEVE, CON   egg shaped meringue, poached in
  vanilla flavored boiling milk, served with custard sauce

LECHE DULCE   sweet, thick cream of boiled milk

LECHE FRITA   fried custard squares

LECHE FRITA CON ANÍS   fried milk custard with flamed
  anisette liqueur

LECHE MERENGADA   cinnamon flavored ice milk

LENGUAS DE GATO   wafer thin crisp cookies served
  with ice cream or custard

LIMA   lime

LIMÓN   lemon

LLAMA   flamed with brandy

LLAMINADURE   pastry, dessert, sweet

MACEDONIA DE FRUTA   fruit salad

MADUIXA   strawberry

MANDARINA   mandarin orange

MANGO   tropical fruit

MANÍ   peanut

MANJAR BLANCO   almond-milk pudding

MANTECADA   sweet dough baked and sprinkled with sugar and cinnamon

MANTECADO   ice cream with frozen whipped cream texture; French ice cream

MANTECADOS   cookies

MANZANA   apple

MANZANA ASADA   baked apple

MANZANA DULCE   apple in honey

MARQUESITAS   chocolate confections made with chopped almonds, sugar and egg yolk

MASITAS   cupcakes

MAZAPÁN   almond paste

MAZAPÁN DE TOLEDO   paste of ground almonds, sugar and egg whites

MEL I MATO   patty of cottage cheese with honey and roasted hazelnuts

MELBA   fruits poached in syrup with vanilla ice cream and raspberry sauce

MELINDRES YEPES   almond marzipan candies

MELOCOTÓN   peach

MELOCOTÓN MELBA   peach poached in syrup with vanilla ice cream and raspberry sauce

MELÓN   melon

MELÓN MIEL, CON   honey melon

MELÓN OPORTO   melon flavored with port wine

MEMBRILLO   quince jelly dessert

MEMBRILLO CON QUESO   quince jelly slice eaten with cheese

MERENGUE   meringue

MERMELADA   jam

MERMELADA DE NARANJA   marmelade, orange jam

MIEL   honey

MIL HOJAS CREMA   pastry layered with custard and frosted on top

MIRABEL   yellow plum

MORA   mulberry

MOUSSE DE CHOCOLATE   frothy chocolate pudding dessert
NARANJA   orange
NATA   cream
NATA BATIDA   whipped cream
NATA MONTADA   whipped cream
NATILLAS   custard
NATILLAS BIZCOCHO, CON   custard over ladyfinger
NATILLAS ESPAÑOLAS   custard over sweet biscuit
NATILLAS LIMÓN, DE   custard with lemon cream
NATILLAS NUECES, CON   soft milk custard with walnuts
NEULE   rolled cookie
NÍSPERO   tart fruit that grows wild
NUECES   nuts
OLIVAS   olives
OMELETTE ALASKA   dessert with ice cream center
    covered with meringue, oven browned and flamed with
    brandy
OMELETTE SURPRISE   Baked Alaska
OVAS MOLES   egg yolk icing
PALTA   avocado
PAN MUNICIÓN   chocolate custard cake with chocolate
    sauce
PAN SANTA TERESA   French toast
PANELLET   marzipan cookie
PANELLETS   Catalán almond cookies
PAPAYA   a tropical fruit
PAPOS ANJO   egg cakes in syrup
PARFAIT   ice cream mixed with egg yolks, cooked and
    cooled, whipped cream and flavorings added, then
    chilled in a mold
PASAS   raisins
PASTAS   pastry
PASTEL HELADO   liquor soaked spongecake with ice cream
PASTEL HOJALDRADO   puff pastry *or* cream puff
PASTEL MANZANA, DE   apple-mint crisp pastry
PASTEL NATA Y CREMA, CON   pastry with whipped
    cream and custard

PASTEL NUECES, CON   pastry with chopped nuts
PASTEL SUIZO   individual pastries sprinkled with sugar
PASTEL YEMA HELADO   pastry made with egg yolk and sugar cream filling, frozen
PASTELERÍA   pastry *or* pastry shop
PASTELERÍA FINA   delicate pastry
PASTELES   cakes
PASTELES FRUTAS, DE   fruit tarts
PASTELES HIGOS, CON   baked puff pastry with fig and candied squash filling
PASTELILLO   little tart
PASTELITOS   small cakes
PASTELS NATA   custard tarts
PEÑASANTA   individual Baked Alaska
PERA   pear
PERA ALMÍBAR, EN   pear in syrup
PERA BELLA ELENA   pear poached in syrup, filled with ice cream, covered with chocolate sauce
PERAS CON VINO   stewed pears in cinnamon and wine sauce
PERO   apple
PESTIÑOS   honey covered fritter
PESTIÑOS ANDALUCES   crullers with lemon and anise liqueur
PESTIÑOS CON ANÍS   licorice flavored fried pastry
PETITSOUS   chocolate eclair
PIGNOLI   pine nuts
PIJAMA   dessert with peaches, pineapple, custard, cake and ice cream
PIÑA   pineapple
PIÑA BANDA   slice of pineapple
PIÑA CONSERVA   canned pineapple
PIÑA MACERADA   crushed pineapple
PIÑA PRALINEE FLAMBÉ   pineapple with caramel, flamed
PIÑÓN   pine nut
PINYÓN   pine nut
PISTACHO   pistachio nut

PLATAN FRITO   fried banana pastry

PLÁTANOS   bananas

PLÁTANOS CON MIEL Y PIÑONES   bananas with honey and pine nuts

PLATO DE FRIVOLIDADES   plate of assorted pastries

POLVORÓN   hazelnut cookie

POLVORONES   cinnamon cookies

POLVORONES SEVILLANOS   brandy flavored butter cookies

POMELO   grapefruit

POMELO KIRSCH   grapefruit with kirsch, a cherry brandy

PONCHE SEGOVIANO   sponge cake soaked in liquor with cream filling

PORTO PUDÍN Y FLAN   Portuguese baked caramel custard

POSTRES   desserts

POUDING   pudding

POUDING DIPLOMÁTICO   dessert with ladyfingers in liqueur, Bavarian cream or custard, apricot jam, glazed fruit soaked in rum or kirsch, and light custard sauce

POUDING FRUTAS, DE   fruit pudding

POUDING PASAS, DE   raisin pudding

PRALINE   roasted almonds cooked in vanilla flavored syrup, caramelized and broken into pieces

PROFITEROLES DE CHOCOLATE   pastry puffs filled with ice cream or custard, covered with chocolate sauce

PUDÍN   pudding

PUDÍN DE MANZANA NATILLAS   apple pudding with custard sauce

PUNTO DE NIEVE   whipped cream with beaten egg whites

QUEIJADAS EVORA   sweet cheese tarts

QUESADA   sweet made with fresh cheese, honey and butter

QUESO BANDEJA, EN   tray of assorted cheese

QUESO, CARRO DE   cheese served from a food cart

QUESO ELEGIR   cheese of your choice

QUESOS SURTIDOS   assorted cheeses

RELÁMPAGOS   pastry like eclair, with filling

REQUESÓN CON MIEL   cottage cheese with honey

ROSCAS   a cookie

ROSQUILLA   doughnut

RUSOS   cake with custard filling cut in squares

SALSA MANZANA, DE   apple sauce

SANDÍA   watermelon

SEMIFRÍOS   frozen dessert of ice cream, candied fruits, nuts

SIERRA NEVADA   ice cream dessert covered with meringue

SORBETE DE CHAMPÁN   champagne sherbet

SORBETE DE TURRÓN   ice milk made with almonds and honey

SULTANAS   raisins

TABLA   cheese board

TARTA   tart *or* pie

TARTA ALMENDRAS, DE   almond cake

TARTA CAPUCHINA   spongecake with custard topping

TARTA CIRUELAS, DE   plums layered with cookies or sponge cake, sprinkled with liquor

TARTA CONVENTO, DE   puff pastry tart with chocolate glaze

TARTA GALLEGA   almond cake

TARTA HELADA   ice cream tart

TARTA HUERTO CURA, DEL   cake with frozen orange custard and orange liqueur

TARTA MANTEQUILLA, DE   cookies or sponge cake spread with a chocolate butter cream filling, meringue, nuts and fruits

TARTA MANZANA, DE   open face apple cake with custard inside

TARTA MIL HOJAS   Napoleon

TARTA NARANJA, CON   orange almond cake with orange syrup

TARTA NORMANDA   cake made with apples

TARTA NUECES, CON   chocolate cake with chopped nuts
TARTA PIÑONES, CON   tart with pine nuts
TARTA PONCHE, CON   layered cake with cream filling
   and chopped almonds
TARTA QUESO, DE   cheesecake
TARTA SANTIAGO   almond cake with almond topping
TARTA YEMAS, CON   cake with liquor soaked sponge-
   cake
TECLA CON YEMA   baked puff pastry horns with
   candied egg yolk filling
TOCINILLO CIELLO   sweet made with egg yolk and
   sugar
TOCINO DE CIELO   rich caramel custard with syrup
   inside
TORONJA   grapefruit
TORRIJAS   French toast
TORRIJAS CON VINO   wine-dipped French toast
TORTA ARROZ LECHE, DE   rice pudding cake
TORTA MOCA, DE   mocha layer cake with rum
TORTAS ACEITE, CON   anise and sesame seed cookies
TOSTADAS   French toast with honey
TOUCINHO CEU   almond cake
TURRÓN   whole almonds mixed with honey and sugar
TURRÓN ALICANTE   hard white almond nougat
TURRONES   almond paste
UVA   grape
UVA PASA   raisin
VAINILLA   vanilla
VARIOS AROMAS   various flavors
XOCOLATA   chocolate
YEMAS   whipped egg yolks and sugar
YEMAS COCO   coconut candies made with brandy
YOGHOURT   yogurt
ZABAGLIONE   soft custard of cooked beaten egg yolks,
   sugar and wine
ZARZAMORA   blackberry

Eggs

CHAMPIÑONES REVOLTILLOS   scrambled eggs and sauteed mushrooms

DUELOS QUEBRANTOS   scrambled eggs with bacon and sausage

ESCALFADOS   poached eggs

ESTRELLADOS   fried eggs

HUEVOS   eggs; also see TORTILLA

HUEVOS A SU GUSTO   eggs prepared to your choice

HUEVOS ALCACHOFAS, CON   eggs with artichoke hearts

HUEVOS ANCHOAS, CON   eggs with anchovies

HUEVOS ATÚN, CON   eggs with tuna fish

HUEVOS BACALAO, CON   eggs with dried codfish

HUEVOS BESAMEL, CON   eggs with white sauce of butter, flour and milk; Bechamel sauce

HUEVOS BUTIFARRA, CON   eggs with sausage

HUEVOS CAZUELA, EN   eggs baked in a casserole

HUEVOS CEBOLLA, CON   eggs with onion

HUEVOS CHAMPIÑONES, CON   eggs with mushrooms

HUEVOS CHORIZO, CON   eggs with paprika flavored sausage

HUEVOS COCIDOS   boiled eggs

HUEVOS COCOTTE   shirred eggs

HUEVOS CON ALLIOLI   garlic mayonnaise with eggs

HUEVOS CREMA, CON   eggs with cream sauce

HUEVOS CUBANOS   fried eggs on rice, topped with fried bananas and tomato sauce

HUEVOS DEL MESÓN   special restaurant preparation of eggs

HUEVOS DUROS   hard cooked eggs

HUEVOS ESCALFADOS   shirred eggs

HUEVOS ESCALFADOS BENEDICTINOS   poached eggs on ham covered toast with Hollandaise sauce or a cream sauce

HUEVOS ESCALFADOS CON CREMA   eggs poached in
cream
HUEVOS ESPAÑOLES   eggs stuffed with tomatoes, with
cheese sauce
HUEVOS ESPÁRRAGOS, CON   eggs with asparagus
HUEVOS ESPEJO   eggs coated with cream and cooked
HUEVOS ESPINACAS, CON   eggs with spinach
HUEVOS FLAMENCOS   eggs on a bed of tomatoes,
chorizo, ham, green beans, fried potatoes, asparagus,
red pepper and peas, in small pieces, put in the oven
HUEVOS FLORENTINOS   eggs with spinach and grated
cheese or cheese sauce
HUEVOS FRITOS   fried eggs
HUEVOS FRITOS AMERICANOS   fried eggs, bacon, ham
and tomato
HUEVOS FRITOS CON AJILLO   eggs fried in olive oil
with garlic and paprika
HUEVOS FRITOS ESPAÑOLES   eggs fried in olive oil
served with sausage, potatoes, croutons
HUEVOS FRITOS HUERTANOS   fried eggs with mixed
vegetables
HUEVOS FRITOS SEVILLANOS   fried eggs with ham,
anchovy stuffed olives, sausage; *or* nests of tomatoes,
onion, garlic and ham with fried egg placed in middle
HUEVOS GELATINA, CON   eggs in aspic
HUEVOS GRAN DUQUESA   poached egg on fried bread
with truffle, cheese sauce and grated cheese, asparagus,
crayfish tails, oven-browned
HUEVOS GRATINADOS   eggs covered with sauce, bread
crumbs, grated cheese and then browned
HUEVOS GUISADOS   eggs fried in olive oil
HUEVOS GUISANTES, CON   eggs with peas
HUEVOS HIGADILLOS DE POLLO, CON   eggs with
chicken livers
HUEVOS HOLANDESES   eggs with cream sauce of egg
yolks, butter and lemon juice
HUEVOS HORNO, AL   baked eggs

HUEVOS LANGOSTINOS   eggs with prawns
HUEVOS LONGANIZA, CON   eggs with sausage
HUEVOS MADRILEÑOS   eggs baked with sausage,
 tomatoes, grated cheese
HUEVOS MAGRA CABALLO   slice of fried ham topped
 with a fried egg
HUEVOS MARISCOS, CON   eggs with seafood
HUEVOS MAYONESA   hard-boiled eggs with mayonnaise
HUEVOS MEYERBEER   eggs with lamb kidney and
 truffle sauce
HUEVOS MIGAS, CON   scrambled eggs with fried bread
 croutons
HUEVOS MOLDEADOS   eggs cooked in a mold
HUEVOS MORCILLA, CON   eggs with blood sausage
HUEVOS MORNAY   eggs with white cream sauce and
 grated cheese
HUEVOS NANTUA   eggs with sauce made using crayfish
 stock
HUEVOS NATURALES   plain eggs
HUEVOS NIDO, EN   egg yolk placed in roll, fried and
 covered with egg white
HUEVOS PARMESANOS   eggs with grated Parmesan cheese
HUEVOS PASADOS POR AGUA   soft-boiled eggs
HUEVOS PATATAS, CON   eggs with potatoes
HUEVOS PICADILLOS CON CHAMPIÑONES   eggs
 baked on top of chopped mushrooms
HUEVOS PIPERADOS VASCOS   scrambled eggs with bell
 peppers, tomatoes, onions and fried ham
HUEVOS PISTO   eggs with cooked vegetables
HUEVOS RELLENOS CON GAMBAS   hard eggs stuffed
 with shrimp
HUEVOS RELLENOS CON SALMÓN   salmon stuffed
 hard eggs
HUEVOS REVUELTOS   scrambled eggs; also see
 TORTLLIAS
HUEVOS RUSOS FRÍOS   cold, stuffed hard-boiled egg
 halves with mayonnaise

HUEVOS SALMORREJO   eggs baked in olive oil, garlic, onion, with ham, pork loin, sausage and asparagus spears

HUEVOS TOCINO, CON   bacon and eggs

OUS   eggs; also see HUEVOS

PIPARRADA   scrambled eggs with tomato, onion, ham, peppers, garlic

PLATO DE HUEVOS   fried eggs

PLATO DE HUEVOS CHASSEUR   fried eggs in pastry shells with chicken livers and tomato-wine sauce with mushrooms

PLATO DE HUEVOS LORRENA   eggs on grilled bacon and Swiss cheese, baked

PLATO DE HUEVOS MALLORQUINA   fried eggs with sausage

PLATO DE HUEVOS MANTECA NEGRA   fried eggs with browned butter

PLATO DE HUEVOS NEGUS   fried eggs on a meat croquette with truffle sauce

PLATO DE HUEVOS ROTHMAGO   eggs on sauteed ham, baked, garnished with sausage and tomato sauce

PLATO DE HUEVOS TURBIGO   fried eggs with sausages and mushrooms or lamb kidney and grilled tomato

PLATO DE HUEVOS TURCA   fried eggs with fried onion rings, chicken livers, tomato sauce

PLATO DE HUEVOS WLADEMIR   cream coated eggs with grated cheese, browned and served with asparagus and truffles

PORTUGUESA   eggs cooked with tomatoes

PRINCESA   eggs cooked with asparagus

RELLENOS   stuffed hard eggs

REVOLTILLO   scrambled eggs; also see HUEVOS

REVUELTOS   scrambled eggs

REVUELTOS AHUMADOS   eggs with smoked meat or fish

REVUELTOS AJETS, CON   eggs soft scrambled with scallions

REVUELTOS CALABICINES, CON   eggs with squash

REVUELTOS CAVIAR, CON   eggs with caviar

REVUELTOS LANGOSTINO Y ESPINACAS, CON   soft scrambled eggs with shrimp and spinach

REVUELTOS MADRILEÑOS   eggs with cream and sauteed tomatoes

REVUELTOS ORLOFF   eggs mixed with cream, crayfish and truffle added

REVUELTOS PERIGUEUX   eggs with truffle sauce

REVUELTOS VASQUERA   sauteed tomatoes and onion with Serrano ham

ROSSINI   eggs with goose liver and Madeira sauce

SOUFFLÉ   baked egg dish with various flavorings or grated ingredients

SOUFFLÉ DE SALMÓN   baked egg dish with salmon

SOUFFLÉ DE SESOS   baked egg dish with sauteed brains

SOUFFLÉ DE ZANAHORIAS   baked egg dish with carrots

TORTILLA   omelette plain or with cheese, ham, mushrooms, chicken livers, seafood filling; also see HUEVOS

TORTILLA ABUELO   omelette with parsley and fried bread cubes

TORTILLA AJITOS SILVESTRES, CON   omelette with young, wild garlic

TORTILLA ALICANTINA   omelette with onion, shrimp, asparagus, ham and tomato

TORTILLA AMPURDANESA   omelette with cooked white beans

TORTILLA ANDALUZA   omelette with sauteed tomatoes, ham, pimiento, mushrooms

TORTILLA ANGUILAS, CON   omelette with fried baby eels

TORTILLA ARANJUEZ   omelette with asparagus tips

TORTILLA ASTURIANA   omelette with tuna fish, onion and tomato

TORTILLA ATÚN ESCABECHADO, DE   omelette with marinated tuna fish and onion

TORTILLA ATÚN, DE   omelette with potatoes, spinach, chunks of tuna

TORTILLA BACALAO, DE   omelette with codfish and onion

TORTILLA BETANZOS   potato omelette

TORTILLA BUENA MUJER   fried bacon, fried onion and mushroom omelette

TORTILLA CATALANA   omelette with sauteed tomatoes, green pepper and eggplant

TORTILLA CHAMPIÑONES, CON   omelette with mushroom, ham, garlic

TORTILLA CHANGET   omelette with fried whitebait fish

TORTILLA COMBINADA   omelette with combination of local ingredients

TORTILLA CONFITURA, CON   jam omelette

TORTILLA CORUÑESA   omelette with potatoes and cured ham

TORTILLA DÁTILES, CON   omelette with shrimp, ham, dates, tomato sauce

TORTILLA DE GRANADA   omelette made with lamb sweetbreads, chicken liver and kidney with white wine

TORTILLA DE SU ELECCIÓN   omelette of your choice

TORTILLA DULCE   jam omelette

TORTILLA ESCABECHE, CON   omelette with pickled fish

TORTILLA ESPAÑOLA   omelette with sliced potatoes and onions fried in oil

TORTILLA ESTRAGÓN, CON   omelette with tarragon

TORTILLA EXTREMEÑA   omelette with sausage and potatoes

TORTILLA FINES DE HIERBAS, CON   omelette with chopped fresh herbs

TORTILLA GAMBAS, CON   omelette with prawns and prawn sauce

TORTILLA GARBANZOS, CON   omelette with chick-peas

TORTILLA HABAS, CON   omelette with lima beans

TORTILLA HÚNGARA   omelette with onions sauteed with ham and paprika cream sauce

TORTILLA JAMÓN, DE   ham omelette

TORTILLA LACÓN, CON   omelette with pork shoulder meat

TORTILLA LEGUMBRES, CON   omelette with mixed, diced, cooked vegetables

TORTILLA LORRENA   omelette with grilled bacon,
  Gruyere cheese, cream and chives mixed in eggs
TORTILLA LYONESA   omelette with sliced fried onions
  and eggs
TORTILLA MAGRA   lean ham omelette
TORTILLA MARINESCA   seafood omelette
TORTILLA MURCIANA   omelette with sauteed tomatoes,
  onions, squash, eggplant
TORTILLA NAVARRA   tomatoes sauteed with garlic,
  eggs on top, with fried sausage, cheese, oven-baked
TORTILLA PAISANA   omelette with ham and vegetables
TORTILLA PATATA ESPAÑOLA, DE   Spanish potato omelette
TORTILLA PATATAS, DE   omelette made with potatoes
  and onions, fried in olive oil
TORTILLA SABOYARDA   eggs mixed with Swiss cheese
  and poured over sauteed potatoes
TORTILLA SESOS, CON   omelette with sauteed brains
TORTILLA SETAS, CON   omelette with wild mushrooms
TRUITA DE PATATA   potato omelette
TRUITA SAMFAINA   mixed vegetable omelette
TURCA   with chicken livers

Fritters and Pancakes

AREPA   corn flapjack
BARTOLILLOS   custard filled fried pastry made with
  wine, lemon peel, cinnamon
BREVAS SORIA   custard filled small doughnuts
BUÑUELITOS CHORIZO   fritters made with chopped
  sausage
BUÑUELITOS DE BACALAO   cod fritters
BUÑUELITOS DE HUEVO DURO   hard-boiled egg fritters
BUÑUELITOS DE JAMÓN   ham fritters
BUÑUELITOS DE POLLO   chicken fritters
BUÑUELO   fritter *or* doughnut
BUÑUELOS   sweet fritters; also see BUNYOL and BUÑUELO
BUÑUELOS CON PLÁTANO   deep fried banana fritters

BUÑUELOS SAN ISIDRO   deep fried sweet fritters
   custard filled
BUÑUELOS VIENTO   deep fried sweet fritters
BUNYOL DE BACALLA   salt cod fritter
BUNYOL DE CIURENY   wild mushroom fritter
CORTADILLO   small pancake
CREPES   thin filled pancake with creamy sauce
CROQUETAS POLLO, DE   chicken croquettes
CROQUETES LLAGOSTA, DE   lobster croquettes
HAYACA CENTRAL   cornmeal pancake with minced
   meat filling
PATATA FRITA   deep fried potato patty
PIOS NONOS   chicken and potato croquettes
ROSQUILLAS RÍO JANAS   small doughnuts made with
   wine, anise and sugar
TORTA   pancake
TORTITA   waffle

Game

BECADA   woodcock
CACA   wild game
CAZA   game
CAZADORA   with mushrooms, onions, wine
CIERVO   deer, venison
CIVET   deer stew with onions and mushrooms
CODORNICES   quail
CODORNICES ASADAS EN HOJAS DE UVA   quail
   baked, wrapped in grape leaves
CODORNICES CEREZAS, CON   braised quail with cherries
CODORNICES ESCABECHE, EN   grilled or roasted quail
   in a marinade
CODORNICES ESTOFADAS   braised quail with onion,
   garlic, wine and brandy
CODORNICES HIDO   quail done in brandy and wine,
   onion, pepper, served in a nest of French fried potatoes
CODORNICES, PAREJA DE   two braised quail in sauce

CODORNICES PERIGOURDINE   quail casserole roasted
with Madeira flavored gravy

CODORNICES POCHAS CALZADAS   quail with lima
beans, onion, tomato, sausage

CODORNICES UVAS, CON   poached quail with peeled
grapes, wine flavored aspic

CODORNICES ZURRÓN   quail wrapped in ham, inside
green pepper with tomatoes and onions

CODORNIZ   quail

CONEJO   rabbit

CONEJO ALIOLI, CON   broiled rabbit, baked in wine
garlic sauce

CONEJO AMPURDANESO   braised rabbit in broth with
onion, tomato and rabbit liver paste, chocolate, garlic,
pepper and almonds

CONEJO CASERO   braised rabbit in wine, onion,
mushrooms, bacon and lard

CONEJO CAZADOR   rabbit casserole, flamed in brandy
with onion, wine, tomato, mushrooms

CONEJO CIRUELAS Y PIÑONES, CON   sauteed rabbit
with prunes and pine nuts

CONEJO JUANA, A LA   baked rabbit with tomatoes,
garlic, onion, olive oil, almonds, cognac

CONEJO, MUSLO DE   roasted rabbit thigh

CONEJO PEPITORIA, A LA   baked rabbit with egg,
lemon sauce and mushrooms

CONEJO ALIOLI, PIERNA DE   broiled rabbit leg with
garlic mayonnaise

CONEJO PIRINEO   rabbit casserole with onion, wine,
pine nuts, almond and garlic

CONEJO SALMANTINO   rabbit potted with onion,
garlic, vinegar, olive oil, pepper

CONEJO SOBRE BRASAS   rabbit broiled over charcoal

CONEJO THEBUSSEM   braised rabbit pieces with a sauce
of oil, bread and ground almonds

CONEJO TOMATE, CON   rabbit marinated in wine,
sauteed in wine, onion, garlic, red pepper

CONEJO VINO BLANCO, CON   rabbit sauteed in butter, simmered in a casserole with white wine

CONILL   rabbit

CORZO   deer

CORZO AUSTRIAZA   roasted deer with caraway seeds

CORZO SOLOMILLO   filet or loin of deer

FAISÁN   pheasant

FAISÁN ALCÁNTARO   pheasant stuffed with liver, wild mushrooms, marinated in port wine and roasted

FAISÁN CREMA, CON   pheasant roasted with onions, served with sauce of roasting juices and cream

FAISÁN SOUVAROFF   pheasant stuffed with sauteed goose liver, roasted in earthenware pot with Madeira wine

FAISÁN UVAS, CON   pheasant poached in veal stock and served cold with wine flavored aspic

GALLINA GUINEA   guinea fowl

GALLO   cockerel rooster *or* black grouse

GAMO   buck

JABALÍ   wild boar

JABALÍ, CABEZA DE   de-boned boar's head with stuffing containing pistachio nuts

JABALÍ EN ADOBO, CHULETAS DE   wild boar chops marinated, grilled or broiled with spicy sauce

JABALÍ, LOMO DE   saddle of boar

JABALÍ, PERNIL DE   haunch of boar

LIEBRE   hare

LIEBRE CIVET   stew of hare with onions and mushrooms

LIEBRE ESTOFADA   jugged hare

LIEBRE FABES   hare braised and stewed with broad beans

MORTERUELO   pork liver, giblets, game and a variety of spices

MUSLO DE CONEJO   roasted rabbit thigh

OCA   goose

OCA CON PERAS   baby roast goose with pine nuts, raisins, pears, wine, with pears caramelized after cooking

PALOMA   dove

PALOMINO   pigeon

PATO SALVAJE ROYAL   roast wild duck
PATO SILVESTRE   wild duck
PERDICES ESTOFADAS   stuffed braised partridges
PERDIZ   partridge
PERDIZ BILBAÍNA   braised partridge with onion, wine,
   cognac, placed on fried bread with pan juice and tomato
   sauce
PERDIZ CASTELLANA   braised partridge with oil, wine,
   vinegar, onion and black pepper
PERDIZ CHOCOLATE, CON   partridge in chocolate
   flavored wine sauce
PERDIZ CROQUETAS COL, CON   baked partridge with
   cabbage croquettes
PERDIZ ENCEBOLLADA   partridge sauteed in oil with
   onions and white wine
PERDIZ ESCABECHADA   partridge braised and marin-
   ated in herb oil and vinegar
PERDIZ ESCABECHE, CON   marinated partridge
PERDIZ ESTOFADO   partridge stewed in wine, onion,
   garlic
PERDIZ ESTRAGÓN, CON   braised partridge in tarragon
   sauce
PERDIZ GUISADA CON COLES   partridge stewed in
   cabbage, braised in broth, tomatoes, onions, peppers
   and oil
PERDIZ JUGO, CON   partridge roasted and served in pan
   juices
PERDIZ TOLEDANA   braised partridge in oil, vinegar,
   garlic, onions, wine
PERDIZ VINAGRETA, A LA   baked partridge in wine
   vinegar sauce
PERDIZ VINO TINTO, CON   braised partridge with oil,
   onions, garlic, tomatoes and wine
PICHÓN   pigeon
PICHÓN CON SALSA   pigeon braised and served in
   onion, tomato, oil, garlic and orange juice
PICHONCILLO   squab

PICHONES   squabs *or* pigeons
PICHONES ESTOFADOS   braised stuffed squabs
PIERNA DE CONEJO CON ALIOLI   broiled rabbit leg
   with garlic mayonnaise
PINTADA   guinea fowl
QUATLLES   quail
TOJUNTO   rabbit, garlic, onion, green pepper, olive oil all
   cooked together
TORDO   thrush
VENADO   venison

Meat

ADOBADO   marinated
ADOBO   marinated
AJIACO   meat and potato stew
ALBÓNDIGAS   pork meatballs
ALBÓNDIGAS MAYONESA   pork meatballs with mayon-
   naise garlic dip
ALBÓNDIGAS SANT CLIMENT   lamb meatballs in rich
   brandy sauce
ALBONDIGÓN   meat loaf
AMBAS SALSAS   two sauces of chef's choice
ARROZ COSTRA   chicken, rabbit, sausages, black pud-
   ding, chick-peas topped with meatballs made of pork,
   hidden under beaten egg, baked in oven to form a crust
ARROZ PARRILLADO   rice, meats, chicken and vegetables
AST   on a spit
BAJOCA FARCIDES   peppers stuffed with rice, pork,
   tomatoes and spices
BIEN COCIDO   steak well-done
BIEN HECHO   well-done
BIEN PASADO   well-done
BIFE PORTUGUÉS   garlic rubbed steak, pan fried in olive
   oil
BIFTEC   steak
BISTEC   beefsteak

BISTEC DE TERNERA   veal steak

BOU   beef

BRASA   cooked over coals

BRASEADO   braised

BROCHETAS   skewered

BUEY   ox

BUTIFARRA Y SETAS   baked sausages and mushrooms

CABEZA DE TERNERA   calf's head

CABRA   goat

CABRITO   kid

CACHOPO   beef stuffed with ham, asparagus tips, breaded and pan fried

CALDERETA   stew of kid goat, fried with piquant peppers and seasoned with mashed liver, raw garlic and red peppers

CALDERETA DE CABRITO   goat stew in red wine

CALLOS   tripe, stomach lining

CALLOS ANDALUZ   tripe stewed in mint sauce, beans, onion, tomato, pimento, ham and sausage

CALLOS ASTURIANOS   tripe stewed with pig's feet, sausage, ham, bell peppers, onion, hot pepper, garlic, tomato paste and oil

CALLOS MADRILEÑOS   tripe in a sauce of tomato, onion with black pudding, chorizo and ham

CARBONADA   meat stew

CARBONADA CRIOLLA   pumpkin stuffed with beef and baked

CARBONADA DE VACA   braised beef in beer with tomato puree

CARNE   meat

CARNE ASADA AL HORNO   roast meat

CARNE CASTELLANA   slices of beef and ham sauteed in onions, garlic, wine and oil

CARNE CERDO, DE   pork

CARNE FUEGO LEÑA   charcoal broiled meats

CARNE MOLIDA   chopped beef

CARNE PARRILLA, A LA   charcoal grilled steak

CARNE PICADA   chopped beef

CARNE TERNERA   veal
CARNE VACA, DE   beef
CARNE VINO   pork braised in white wine
CARNERO   mutton
CASTELLÓN DE OLLA   stew of white beans, beef and bacon
CATALANA   with onions, parsley and tomatoes
CAZADORA   with mushrooms, onions, wine
CAZOULET TOLOSANA   casserole with white beans,
   pork, ham, fresh bacon, sausages and duck meat
CAZUELA DE CORDERO   lamb stew with vegetables
CAZUELA DE LOMO BUTIFARRA   pork chops and
   sweet sausage casserole
CEBOLLAS RELLENAS   beef stuffed onions with wine,
   cream and cheese
CEBÓN   castrated beef
CERDO   pork
CERDO CARRE   bone-in pork loin roast
CERDO, CHULETAS DE   pork chops
CERDO, CINTA DE   loin of pork
CERDO CORTIJERA, A LA   pork braised in olive oil
CERDO ESTERHAZY, FILETE DE   pork browned, pap-
   rika seasoned, simmered in sour cream
CERDO, FILETE DE   pork tenderloin
CERDO, LOMO DE   pork loin
CERDO, LONJA DE   pork loin or pork chop, pan fried
CERDO, MANITAS DE   pigs' feet breaded and pan fried
CERDO, NORMANDA, A LA   pork chops in sauce from
   pan juices with cream
CERDO, OLLA DE   pork loin fried in earthenware pot
CERDO ORÉGANO, CON   pork cooked with oregano
CERDO PORTUGUÉS   pork slices coated with garlic paste
   and browned in white wine and broth
CERDO PROVENZALE, A LA   pork loin seasoned with
   sage and roasted with garlic and olive oil
CERDO RIOJANA, A LA   pork with tomatoes and bell
   peppers
CERDO SARTÉN, EN   roasted pork loin sauteed in butter

CERDO, SOLOMILLO DE   pork tenderloin
CHANCHO ADOBADO   pork, sweet potatoes, orange
    and lemon juice
CHANFAINA   goat liver and kidney stew in thick sauce
CHANFAINA SALMANTINA   dish of rice, giblet, lamb
    sweetbread and pieces of chorizo
CHATEAUBRIAND   steak from center of filet
CHATEAUBRIAND BUEY MASCOTA   steak sauteed
    with wine and sauce made from pan juices
CHORIZO   sausage of pork, pork fat, spices, herbs and
    paprika
CHOTO   bull meat
CHULETAS   cutlets
CHULETAS AÑONO   mutton chops
CHULETAS CARNERO   lamb *or* mutton chop
CHULETAS CASTELLANA   veal chops browned in lard
CHULETAS CORDERO PARISIENNE, DE   lamb chops
    grilled with browned potatoes, artichoke bottoms,
    Madeira sauce
CHULETAS DE CERDO   pork chops
CHULETAS DE CERDO ASTURIANAS   pork chops with
    apples in cider sauce
CHULETAS DE CERDO CON CIRUELA PASA   pork
    chops, prunes, cinnamon, wine
CHULETAS DE CERDO CON JEREZ   pork chops with
    sherry and almonds
CHULETAS DE CERDO CON PIMIENTOS JAMÓN   pork
    chops sauteed with pimientos, ham, tomato, onions
CHULETAS DE CERDO RIOJANA   pork chops sauteed
    with pimientos, tomato, onions
CHULETAS DE CORDERO   lamb chops
CHULETAS DE CORDERO A LA NAVARRA   lamb chops
    and sausages in tomato sauce
CHULETAS DE CORDERO CON ALLIOLI   grilled rib
    lamb chops with garlic mayonnaise
CHULETAS DE CORDERO ROMESCO   grilled rib lamb
    chops with peppery sauce

CHULETAS DE CORDERO VILLEROI   lamb fried with brown meat sauce, breaded and fried again
CHULETAS DE PUERCO   pork chops
CHULETAS DE TERNASCO   baby lamb chops
CHULETAS DE TERNERA   veal cutlets
CHULETAS DE TERNERA AJO CABINIL   veal chops sauteed with garlic, vinegar and paprika
CHULETAS DE TERNERA CAZUELA   veal chops braised in sauce with oil, tomatoes and onion
CHULETAS DE TERNERA CON HABAS   veal chops with lima beans in onion, tomato sauce
CHULETAS DE TERNERA HORTELANAS   veal chops with ham, mushrooms and finely chopped vegetables
CHULETAS HOLSTEIN   veal cutlets topped with egg
CHULETAS PAPILLOTE   cutlets sauteed in butter with chopped mushrooms, sealed in paper and oven baked
CHULETAS VILLAGODIO   rib steak with bone in
CHULETAS ZINGARA, A LA   cutlets sauteed in butter with Marsala wine and mushroom sauce
CHULETÓN   large rib steak
CHURRASCO   charcoal grilled meat, generally beef
COCHIFRITO   fricassee of lamb
COCHIFRITO DE CORDERO   lamb or kid stew
COCHIFRITO NAVARRO   small pieces of fried lamb
COCHINILLO   roast pig
COCHINILLO ASADO   roast suckling pig
COCHINILLO SEGOVIANO   suckling pig in clay oven, baked with wine
COCIDO   a boiled dinner of soup, vegetables, meat, bacon, black pudding, chick-peas
COCIDO ANDALUZ   beef, pork, sausage, squash, green beans, garlic cooked into a soup-stew
COCIDO MADRILEÑO   a soup-stew of chick-peas, veal or beef, ham, salt pork, potatoes, sausage, cabbage, chicken, carrots, onions, pig's feet and garlic
COCIDO PORTUGUÉS   boiled meats, chicken and vegetables
COLA   tail

COLA ANDALUZA   braised tail with potatoes, onion, garlic, tomato

COLA DE TORO   bull's tail braised in gravy with onion, cabbage, carrots, bacon and sausage

CONEJO   rabbit

CONILL   rabbit

CONTRA FILETE   boneless loin of beef

CONTRA TERNERA   veal loin steak

CORAZONADA   heart stew

CORDERO   lamb

CORDERO ASADO   baby lamb roasted over coals

CORDERO ASADO CASTELLANO   oven roasted lamb with garlic, onion, cumin, oregano

CORDERO ASADO MANCHEGO   roast lamb with garlic, cognac, olive oil, black pepper

CORDERO ASADO SEPULVEDANO   roast lamb in garlic vinegar wine sauce

CORDERO, BRAZUELO DE   roasted front leg of lamb

CORDERO, CALDERETA DE   lamb stew

CORDERO, CHULETAS DE   lamb chops; also see CHULETAS

CORDERO CHILINDRÓN   fried lamb chunks with peppers and tomatoes

CORDERO VILLEROI, CHULETAS DE   fried lamb chops with brown meat sauce, breaded and fried again

CORDERO CHULETAS GUÉRNICA   breaded and pan fried lamb chops

CORDERO CHULETAS NAVARRA   lamb chops sauteed then braised in tomato sauce and onion

CORDERO CHULETAS PARISIENNE   grilled lamb chops with browned potatoes, artichoke bottoms, Madeira sauce

CORDERO COCHIFRITO   sautee of lamb with garlic and lemon

CORDERO, COSTILLAS DE   lamb rib chops

CORDERO, ESPALDA DE   roasted boned and stuffed lamb shoulder

CORDERO GUISADO   lamb stew

CORDERO LECHAL   milk-fed lamb
CORDERO, MANITAS DE   stewed lamb's feet
CORDERO MENESTRA   lamb and vegetable soup-stew
CORDERO MENUDILLOS   lamb's internal organs, sauteed
CORDERO PASCUAL   mutton
CORDERO, PATA DE   roasted leg of lamb
CORDERO RECENTAL   spring lamb
CORDERO RIOJANA   stewed with pepper, tomato, garlic
  and oil
CORDON BLEU   slices of veal, slice of ham and Swiss
  cheese, breaded and fried
CORONA CORDERO   crown of lamb
COSTELETA   cutlet; also see CHULETAS
COSTILLA   lamb rib or chop; also see CHULETAS
COSTILLA DE ADÁN   charcoal broiled beef rib steak
COSTILLA DE CORDERO   lamb chop
COSTILLA GALLEGA   broiled veal chop
COSTILLAS DE CERDO   spareribs
CRIADILLAS DE TORO   bull testicles
CROQUETAS   meat, fish or vegetable croquettes
CUCHIFRITO   milk-fed suckling pig
CURANTO   seafood, vegetables and pig cooked in an
  earthen well
DON SUERO   ham stuffed veal cutlet
EN SU JUGO   in its own juice
ENTRECOTE   boneless beef rib steak
ENTRECOTE ANGLAISE   bonless beef rib steak grilled
  with bacon and potatoes
ENTRECOTE BORDALES   rib steak pan fried in sauce of
  juices, shallots, bone marrow and wine
ENTRECOTE CEBÓN, DE   rib steak from fattened steer
ENTRECOTE CECILIA   beef grilled with mushroom,
  creamed green asparagus tips and puffed potato chips
ENTRECOTE FAVORITO   beef tenderloin pan fried with
  sauteed goose liver
ENTRECOTE GUARNICIÓN, DE   grilled or pan fried
  beef

ENTRECOTE HOSTAL   beef tenderloin pan fried with sauce from boiled down pan juices, wine and meat

ENTRECOTE MARCHAND VINS   beef tenderloin grilled and covered with wine and meat concentrate sauce

ENTRECOTE PIMIENTA   steak with crushed peppercorns, pan fried in butter, served in sauce of pan juices, butter, shallots and cognac

ENTRECOTE PIZZAIOLA   beef tenderloin pan fried with pan juices, garlic, tomatoes and oregano in oil

ENTRECOTE QUESO Y CABRALES, CON   boneless beef tenderloin sauteed with blue cheese, wine, garlic

ENTRECOTE TIROLESA   broiled beef with French fried onion rings

ESCALOPE   boneless meat, usually veal

ESCALOPE BOLOGNÉS   veal breaded, fried with ham and Parmesan cheese, oven melted

ESCALOPE EN CACEROLA   sauteed veal in earthenware dish with sauce from pan juices

ESCALOPE GUÉRNICA   veal breaded and fried in olive oil

ESCALOPE HOLSTEIN   veal pan fried, topped with a fried egg

ESCALOPE MARSALA   veal fried in oil, served in sauce from pan juices and Marsala wine

ESCALOPE MILANÉS   veal dipped in egg, bread crumbs, grated Parmesan cheese and fried

ESCALOPE NAPOLITANO   veal sauteed in butter, coated with sauce, grated cheese, breaded and fried

ESCALOPE NARANJA, CON   veal sauteed in oil, butter and orange juice

ESCALOPE VIENÉS   veal breaded and fried with anchovy butter

ESCALOPE ZÍNGARO   veal sauteed in butter, Marsala wine, mushrooms and served in sauce from pan juices

ESCALOPINES MADRILEÑOS   veal medallions in onion tomato sauce

ESCUDELLA PAYES   soup-stew of meats, sausage, cabbage, garbanzo beans, potatoes, vegetables

ESPALDA   shoulder
ESPÁRRAGOS MONTAÑESES   asparagus with calves'
    tails
ESTOFADO   stew
ESTOFADO BOU   beef stew
ESTOFADO CIRUELAS Y PIÑONES, CON   beef stew
    with prunes and pine nuts
ESTOFADO PATATAS, CON   beef stew with potatoes
ESTOFADO TORO, DE   stew of bull meat, onion, garlic,
    tomatoes, wine, cognac
ESTOFADO VACA, DE   beef stew
FABADA   pork, bean, bacon and sausage stew
FABADA ASTURIANA   stew of large white beans, with ham
    or bacon, sausage, salt pork, onions, garlic and saffron
FARCELLETS   cabbage dumplings *or* rolled meat
FARCELLETS COL   pork and cabbage dumplings
FETGE   calf's liver
FETGE CEBA   calf's liver with onion
FIAMBRES   cold cuts of meat
FIAMBRES SURTIDOS   assorted meat cold cuts
FIAMBRES VARIADOS   assorted meat cold cuts
FIDEOS DE CAZUELA   noodles with spareribs, sausages,
    ham and bacon
FILETE   steak
FILETE BUEY   steer
FILETE EMPANADO   skillet fried breaded beef steak
FILETE HORTELANO   steak served with fresh vegetables
FILETE LOMO, DE   tenderloin steak
FILETE MECHADO   wrapped with pork fat and roasted
FILETE PARRILLA, A LA   grilled steak
FILETE RES, DE   beefsteak
FILETE STROGANOFF   beef cooked in sour cream gravy
    with onions and mushrooms
FILETE TERNERA, DE   veal tenderloin
FILETE VEDELLA SAMFAINA, DE   roast veal filet with
    mixed vegetables
FILETE VEDELLA, DE   roast veal filet

FLAMENCA   with green peppers, onions, tomatoes, peas and sausage

FLAMENQUINES   pork and ham slices fried and served in white sauce

FLAN PEUADA, DE   pigs' feet mousse

FONDUE BORGOÑA   cubes of beef that you cook at table using a long fork and dipping them into a pot of boiling oil

FREGINAT   white beans with fried pork liver

FRICADELAS   ground beef patties pan fried with sherry on fried French bread

FRICANDO   braised veal with wild mushrooms, pork, onion in tomato sauce

FRIJOLADA   bean stew with meats and vegetables

FRITE   pieces of a lamb yearling fried with paprika

FRITURA MIXTA   deep-fried meats, chicken, vegetables or fish

GUISADO   stew

GUISADO ESPAÑOL   stew with beef, olive oil, onions

HAMBURGUESA   hamburger

HAMBURGUESA LIONESA   hamburger with onion, pan fried with pan juices, wine and butter

HAMBURGUESA TIROLIENNE   hamburger pan fried with fried onion rings

HERVIDO   beef and vegetable stew

HÍGADO   liver

HÍGADO CON AJO CABANIL   calves' liver sauteed in wine vinegar, garlic, paprika

HÍGADO CON CEBOLLAS   liver and onions

HÍGADO ENCEBOLLADO   liver sauteed with onions, peppers, wine

HÍGADO INGLÉS   thin slices of liver, coated in flour, fried in butter

HÍGADO LIONÉS   liver fried in butter with onions and a sauce from pan juices

HÍGADO PIMENTOS, CON   calves' liver pan fried in onions and peppers

HOJALDRA   puff pastry used for dessert or with fillings of meat and fish

HOJAS DE PARRA RELLENAS   meat stuffed grape leaves stewed in tomato sauce

HUESO   bone

IGLESIA   underdone; boiled; with boiled vegetables

ISCATÓN   marinated liver with red wine sauce

JAMÓN   ham, mostly air-dried and cured

JAMÓN AGUADILLA   roast fresh ham

JAMÓN BIGARADE   boiled, baked, served in Madeira wine sauce with orange juice

JAMÓN COCIDO   boiled ham

JAMÓN CRUDO   cold, boiled ham

JAMÓN DULCE   ham boiled and served cold

JAMÓN GALLEGO   thinly sliced smoked ham

JAMÓN HUEVO HILADO, CON   boiled ham with egg and sugar mixture coating

JAMÓN OPORTO, CON   boiled ham, baked in a port wine butter sauce

JAMÓN PEPINILLOS, CON   cold boiled ham with pickles

JAMÓN SERRANO   dried ham

JAMÓN YORK   boiled ham

JARDINERA   with carrots, peas and mixed vegetables

JARRETE   veal or lamb shank

JUDÍAS OREJA PIE CERDO   stew of white beans, pig's ears and feet in onion, garlic, tomato gravy

JULIANNA   shredded vegetables

LACÓN   pork shoulder

LACÓN CURADO   salted pork

LECHAL   milk fed veal

LECHECILLAS   sweetbreads

LECHÓN   suckling pig

LENGUA   tongue

LENGUA GELATINA, CON   tongue in aspic

LENGUA PORTUGUESA   tongue braised in tomato, onion, oil

LENGUA SEVILLANA   tongue with green olives, potatoes, red peppers

LIEBRE   hare

LIEBRE ESTOFADA   jugged hare

LLOM   loin of pork

LOMBARDA RELLENA   baked sausage stuffed red cabbage

LOMO   loin, usually pork

LOMO ADOBADO   loin of pork marinated and roasted with lard and potatoes

LOMO CERDO ARAGONÉS, DE   loin of pork with onions and white wine

LOMO CERDO ESCALIBADO, DE   roast pork with eggplant, red and green peppers

LOMO CERDO ZARAGOZANO, DE   pork chops with tomato sauce and black olives

LOMO, CINTA DE   boned loin of pork

LOMO EMBUCHADO   stuffed loin

LOMO MONTADITO   pork loin on a slice of bread

LOMO PUERCO CON PIMIENTOS VERMELHOS DUCES, DE   pork loin with sweet red peppers

LOMO RELLENO SALCHICHA   sausage wrapped in pork slices, sauteed with onion, garlic, wine

LONJA   slice of meat

MADEJAS   lamb intestines wrapped around garlic and roasted

MADRILEÑA   with sausage, tomatoes and paprika

MAGRAS   thick slice of lean ham fried in lard or butter, with tomatoes and vegetables

MAGRAS CON TOMATE   slices of slightly fried ham dipped in tomato sauce

MAGRAS ESTILO ARAGÓN   cured ham in tomato sauce

MANDONGUILLE   meatball

MANITAS   lamb's feet

MANOS   pig's feet

MANOS DE CERDO RELLENAS   stuffed pigs' feet

MATAMBRE   beef rolled and stuffed with vegetables

MIXTO GRILL   mixed grilled meat

MOLLEJA   gizzard
MOLLEJAS   sweetbreads
MOLLEJAS CAZADORA   sweetbreads braised in wine,
    mushrooms, shallots, tomato paste
MOLLEJAS JEREZ, CON   sweetbreads sauteed and
    served in sauce of pan juices and sherry
MOLLEJAS PROVENZALE   fried slices of sweetbreads
    with tomato sauce, anchovies, wine and oil
MOLLEJAS REBOZO, DE   sweetbread slices coated in
    batter and deep fried
MOLLEJAS VINO MADEIRA   sweetbreads with Madeira
    sauce, pan juices and mushrooms
MORCILLO   veal shank
MORRO   pig snout
MORRO ANDALUZ   pig snout stewed in sauce of mint,
    beans, onion, tomato, pimento, ham and chorizo
MORTERUELO   pork liver, giblets, game and a variety of
    spices
MORUNA   pork in barbecue sauce
OLLA   stew *or* soup
OLLA PODRIDA   stew of ham, chick-peas, cabbage,
    leeks, tomatoes, chorizo
OLLITA   pot used for stew; stew
OSSO BUCCO   veal shank braised in onion, garlic, tomato
OVEJA   ewe
PABELLÓN CRIOLLO   beef in tomato sauce with beans,
    rice and bananas
PAELLA   stew of pork, rice, chicken, clams, shrimp
PARRILLA   grilled over an open fire
PARRILLA DE GERONA   veal steak
PARRILLA MIXTA   mixed grill
PARRILLADA INGLESA   mixed grill
PARRILLADA MIXTA   mixed grill
PASADO   done, cooked
PASTEL   baked puff pastry pie sometimes with sausage,
    ham, peppers and onion or a meat loaf

PASTEL CIERVA   pie made with veal, chorizo, hard egg, brains and minced meat in pastry and baked

PASTORA   lamb and vegetable stew

PATA   foot

PATA DE CERDO COCIDA   pickled pork (pig's foot)

PATAS DE CERDO   pigs' feet

PATAS DE CERDO DUROC   poached pigs' feet with brown beef sauce

PATAS DE CERDO EN BRETONA   stewed pigs' feet in tomato sauce with white beans

PECHO TERNERA, DE   breast of veal

PELOTA   fried meat dumplings

PELOTAS   meatballs

PELOTAS COCIDAS   stew of meat wrapped in cabbage leaves, chicken, pork bacon, chick-peas, potatoes

PEPITORIA   stew with onions, green peppers and tomatoes

PERDICES AL CAPELLÁN   sauteed veal slices with ham, salami, garlic, olive oil, wine

PICADILLO   meat mixed with diced fried potatoes; hash

PIERNA   leg

PIERNA DE CORDERO   leg of lamb

PIERNA DE CORDERO AL HORNO   oven roasted leg of lamb

PIMIENTOS CALABACINES RELLENOS   meat stuffed peppers and zucchini, baked

PINCHITOS CARNE   pork marinated and broiled on a skewer

PINCHO MORUNO   seasoned pork cubes grilled on a skewer

POCO HECHO   rare

POCO PASADO   rare

POMES FARCIDES   pork stuffed apples

POTE   meat and vegetable soup-stew

POTE ASTURIANO   stew of cabbage, pig's foot, sausages, bacon, ham and white beans

POTE GALLEGO   stew of pork shoulder, white beans, potatoes, sausages, tomatoes, turnip greens, veal and chicken

PUERCO   pork

PUERCO ESTOFADO   spicy pork stew

PUNTO   medium

RABO   tail

RABO DE TORO ANDALUZ   oxtail stew with wine, onion, ham

RAGÚ   stew *or* fricassee

RELLENO   chopped meat *or* a stuffed preparation

RIÑONES   kidneys

RIÑONES BROCHETA, EN   kidneys grilled on a skewer

RIÑONES COÑAC, CON   kidneys sauteed in sauce of pan juices and cognac

RIÑONES EN BROCHETA   veal kidneys on skewers with mushrooms, ham and bacon

RIÑONES ENSARTADOS   kidneys skewered with ham and bacon, broiled with butter

RIÑONES JEREZ, CON   kidneys in sherry wine

RIÑONES MADEIRA   kidneys sauteed with sauce from pan juices and Madeira

RIÑONES MOSTAZA, CON   kidneys sauteed in sauce from pan juices and mustard

RIÑONES PLANCHA, A LA   grilled kidneys

RIÑONES TURBIGO   sauteed on fried bread with sausages, mushrooms and pan juice, wine and tomato paste sauce

ROJOS COMINO   braised pork with cumin

ROMANA   dipped in batter and fried

ROPA VIEJA   meat hash

ROSBIF   roast beef

RUSTIDO   roast

RUSTIDO CATALANA   veal roast with rum, wine, garlic, pepper

SALCHICHA HIGOS AGRI-DULCES, CON   sausages with sweet and sour figs

SALMI   meat in wine-liqueur sauce with fried bread spread with meat paste

SAN JACOBO   veal cutlet, ham slice, pork cutlet, breaded and pan-fried together

SCHABISCH CAUCASIANA   marinated lamb on skewer with tomato, onion, pepper and grilled

SESOS   brains

SESOS MANTECA NEGRA, CON   brains sauteed in browned butter

SESOS MOLINERA, A LA   brains floured and fried in butter

SESOS REBOZO   brains battered and deep-fried

SESOS ROMANA, A LA   brains floured and breaded and pan-fried

SOLOMILLO   filet *or* entrecote

SOLOMILLO ALL PEBRE   beef roast in a pepper garlic sauce

SOLOMILLO CASADOR   entrecote sauteed in butter in sauce of pan juices, wine, mushrooms

SOLOMILLO DIPLOMÁTICO   whole filet, larded, marinated in wine, pan roasted and served with a sauce from pan juices and wine

SOLOMILLO ESPAÑOL   larded whole filet, pan fried in oil with a sherry gravy with onion, garlic, and oregano

SOLOMILLO HORTELANO   filet sauteed in earthenware pot in sauce from pan juices and butter

SOLOMILLO MAÎTRE D'HÔTEL   grilled steaks with creamed butter and lemon juice

SOLOMILLO PARRILLA, A LA   charcoal broiled steaks

SOLOMILLO PIEMONTESE   filet fried in tomato sauce with pan juices

SOLOMILLO PRUSIANA   steak on charcoal broiler

SOLOMILLO WELLINGTON   whole tenderloin covered with sauteed mushrooms and cooked vegetables in pastry dough

STEAK DIANA   pan fried in creamy pepper sauce

STEAK TARTAR   raw ground beef with raw egg, chopped onions and capers

SU PUNTO   medium

SURTIDOS FIAMBRES   cold meat slices

TABURETE   steak fried in olive oil

TAJADA DE ESTOFADO   fricassee

TAJADA DE FILETE   filet

TAJADA DE HÍGADO   liver

TAJADA DE PICADILLO   knuckle

TAJADA DE RIÑÓN   kidneys

TAJADA DE SESOS   brains

TERNASCO   baby lamb

TERNASCO ASADO   roasted baby lamb

TERNASCO ASADO ARAGONÉS   baby lamb roasted over coals

TERNASCO, CABEZA ASADA DE   roasted baby lamb's head

TERNASCO, COSTILLAS DE   baby lamb chops

TERNASCO PASTORA, A LA   braised in pepper, clove, garlic, vinegar and white wine, milk, oil and potatoes

TERNERA   veal

TERNERA ASADA   oven roasted veal leg

TERNERA BRASEADA   roast veal with pan juice and tomato sauce, with spinach cakes

TERNERA, CABEZA DE   boned and poached veal head

TERNERA, CALDERETA DE   potted roast veal leg

TERNERA CHOP INGLESA   breaded chops fried in butter

TERNERA CON BLANQUETA   veal stew in white herb gravy

TERNERA CONDESITA   veal with sherry

TERNERA EN AGUJA   veal in baked pastry

TERNERA, ESCALOPE DE   veal cutlet

TERNERA ESTOFADA   veal stew

TERNERA EXTREMEÑA   sauteed veal with sausage, green peppers, sherry

TERNERA, FALDA DE   veal flank steak

TERNERA EMPANADOS, FILETES DE   breaded veal cutlets pan fried in olive oil

TERNERA CATALÁN, FRICOANDO DE   veal stew with onion, tomato, mushrooms and wine

TERNERA GRANADINAS, CON   thick cutlets of top round larded with pork fat

TERNERA GUISADA   stewed veal

TERNERA GUISANTES, CON   roast veal with green peas

TERNERA HIGADO, CON   veal liver

TERNERA JARDINERA   roasted veal with cooked fresh vegetables and a sauce of pan juices and pureed vegetables

TERNERA, LENGUA DE   veal tongue slices

TERNERA MADRILEÑA   ham slice between two veal cutlets that are floured and pan fried

TERNERA, MANO DE   calf's foot

TERNERA MECHADA   veal larded with pork, bacon fat or ham

TERNERA MEDALLÓN VICTORIA   sauteed meat served on a chicken croquette with fried tomato

TERNERA MENESTRA, Y   veal and vegetable soup-stew

TERNERA, MOLLEJAS DE   sweetbreads

TERNERA MORCILLO   veal shank

TERNERA PASTEL   veal pâté

TERNERA, PECHO DE   roasted, stuffed and rolled breast of veal

TERNERA, PEZ DE   bottom round of veal

TERNERA, PICADILLO DE   veal hash

TERNERA, PINCHOS DE   veal cubes, marinated, skewered and grilled

TERNERA, PULPETAS DE   veal cutlets with a meat paste spread, rolled, breaded and fried

TERNERA REDONDO ASADO   bottom round roast veal

TERNERA RIOJANA, CON   veal stew with wine, lard, bacon and pigs' feet with tomato puree

TERNERA, ROLLO DE   breaded veal loaf with ham, onion, almond paste, oven-braised

TERNERA SALTEADA CASERA   veal braised with wine and vegetables in brown tomato gravy

TERNERA SEVILLANA   sauteed veal with sherry

TERNERA, SOLOMILLO DE   tenderloin steak

TERNERA TRUFADA   loin spread with veal paste, bacon, ham, truffles, rolled up and poached

TERNERA, ZANCARRON DE   braised veal foot

TESTÍCULOS TORO ALLI I JULIVERT   bull testicles with garlic and parsley

TOCINO   bacon

TORO   bull

TORO, COLA DE   bull's tail

TORO LIDIA   fighting bull

TORO, RABO DE   bull's tail

TORTAS CARNE, DE   meat patties

TORTILLA DE GRANADA   omelette made with lamb sweetbreads, chicken liver and kidney with white wine

TOSTÓN   spit roasted young suckling pig

TOURNEDOS   steak from middle of the filet

TOURNEDOS ALEXANDRA   steak sauteed with sliced truffles

TOURNEDOS BAYANA   steak pan fried and covered with tomato sauce

TOURNEDOS BEATRIX   steak pan fried with sauteed morel mushrooms, artichoke hearts, potatoes, with brown meat sauce

TOURNEDOS BILBAÍNA   steak marinated in oil with garlic paste, breaded and broiled

TOURNEDOS BOUQUETIERE   grilled steak with fresh vegetables

TOURNEDOS BRUXELLOISE   steak pan fried in butter with Madeira sauce from pan juices, served with Brussels sprouts, endive and potatoes

TOURNEDOS CAZADORES   steak pan fried in brown wine sauce with mushrooms, shallots and tomato paste

TOURNEDOS COSTA VASCA, DE   steak sauteed and topped with tomatoes

TOURNEDOS EMPERADOR, AL   steak pan fried with truffle, Madeira sauce

TOURNEDOS ENRIQUE IV, AL   steak pan fried on fried
   bread with artichoke bottom stuffed with butter, wine
   and tarragon sauce

TOURNEDOS ESPAÑOLES   steak pan fried with fried
   sliced onions, grilled tomatoes, rice pilaf with peppers

TOURNEDOS FAVORITOS   steak sauteed with goose
   liver and truffle

TOURNEDOS FINANCIEROS   pan fried steak with
   brown meat sauce

TOURNEDOS MARISCALA, A LA   steak sauteed and
   topped with truffle with concentrated meat gelatin
   glaze

TOURNEDOS MASCOTA, A LA   steak sauteed in
   earthenware with brown sauce from pan juices, wine
   and veal gravy

TOURNEDOS POMPADOUR, A LA   steak sauteed with
   truffle slice, truffle flavored brown sauce

TOURNEDOS RICHELIEU   pan fried or grilled steak

TOURNEDOS ROSSINI   steak pan fried in butter, laid on
   fried bread with slice of fried goose liver, with Madeira
   and pan juice sauce

TRIPAS   tripe, stomach lining of a cow

TRIPAS CATALANA   tripe stewed with wine, tomato,
   pine nuts, almonds, garlic

TRIPAS PORTO   tripe stew

TROUXA VITELA   veal roast with red onion

TUÉTANO TOSTADA   bone marrow poached and served
   on fried bread

VACA   beef

VACA SALADA   corned beef

VALENCIANA   with rice, tomatoes and garlic

VEDELLA   veal

VELDELLA PERES   roast veal loin with pears

VILLAGODIO DE VACA   large rib steak of beef

VIZCAÍNA   with green peppers, tomatoes, garlic

XAI   lamb

ZANCARRÓN VASCO   braised veal foot with ham, sliced
   sausage, fried onions, peppers, tomatoes and broth
ZORZA   chorizo sausage meat

Potatoes

BATATA   sweet potato
BATATAS PORTUGUESA   Portuguese fried potatoes
CACHUELOS   boiled diced potatoes, cabbage, garlic,
   bacon, chorizo sausage
CAMOTE   sweet potato
ENSALADA PATATAS, DE   boiled potato salad
MOJETE   potatoes sauteed with garlic, paprika, tomato
   and bay leaf, with poached egg added
ÑOQUIS   dumplings of potatoes, boiled with a sauce of
   butter and grated cheese, oven browned
PAPAS   South American potatoes
PAPAS ARRUGAS, CON   potatoes baked in their jackets
PAPAS FRITAS   South American fried potatoes
PAPAS HUANCAÍNA   potatoes, cheese and green peppers
PATATA FRITA   deep fried potato patty
PATATAS   potatoes
PATATAS ASADAS   baked potatoes
PATATAS COCIDAS   boiled potatoes
PATATAS FRITAS   French fried potatoes
PATATAS SALSA VERDE, CON   potatoes in green parsley
   sauce
PATATAS SALTEADAS   fried potatoes
PATATE ALLIOLI   potato with olive oil and garlic
PATATE CATALANA   stuffed potato
PATATE RABASSOLE   potato with mushroom
PATATES   potatoes
PATATES ASADOS   roasted potatoes
PATATES ASADOS RELLENOS   stuffed baked potatoes
   with ham
PATATES BRAVOS   potato cubes in thick spicy tomato
   pepper sauce

PATATES CHORIZO, CON   potato cubes with sausage
   and bacon bits
PATATES COCIDOS   boiled potatoes
PATATES DORADOS   fried potatoes
PATATES FRITOS   deep fried potatoes
PATATES JUDÍAS VERDES, CON   potato and green bean
   casserole
PATATES NUEVOS   new potatoes
PATATES PAJA, DE   deep fried shoestring potatoes
PATATES PICANTES   potato slices sauteed with chili
   pepper, garlic and oil
PATATES POBRES   potato slices pan fried in garlic olive
   oil
PATATES, PURÉ DE   mashed potatoes
PATATES RELLENOS   stuffed potatoes
PATATES SALSA VERDE, CON   potato slices sauteed
   with oil, garlic and pepper
PATATES VAPOR, AL   steamed potatoes
PURÉ PAPAS, DE   mashed potatoes
PURÉ PATATAS, DE   mashed potatoes
TRUITA DE PATATA   potato omelet
TUMBET   cake of potato and fried eggplant, covered with
   tomato sauce and peppers, then boiled
YAUTIA   sweet potato

Poultry

ADOBO   marinated
ANDRAJOS   giblets
ARROZ COSTRA   chicken, rabbit, sausages, black pud-
   ding, chick-peas topped with meatballs made of pork,
   hidden under beaten egg, baked in oven to form a crust
ARROZ PARRILLADO   rice, meats, chicken and vegetables
ARROZ, PATO CON   roast duck with sausage and ham
   flavored rice
AVE   bird
AVE SUPREMA   boneless breast of chicken

AVE SUPREMA PERIGOT   chicken breasts stuffed with truffle flavored veal paste, poached in butter

AVES   poultry

CAPÓN   castrated roaster chicken

CAPÓN SOUVAROFF   roast stuffed with goose liver, braised in pastry

CATALANA   with onions, parsley and tomatoes

COCIDO PORTUGUÉS   boiled meats, chicken and vegetables

CROQUETAS DE GALLINA   chicken croquettes

CROQUETAS POLLO, DE   chicken croquettes

ESCABECHE GALLINA   chicken marinated in vinegar

FLAMENCA   with green peppers, onions, tomatoes, peas and sausage

FRITURA MIXTA   deep-fried meats, chicken, vegetables or fish

GALLINA   hen

GALLINA CON GARBANZOS   chicken stewed with chick-peas

GALLINA CON SALSA DE ALMENDRAS   stewed chicken in almond wine sauce

GALLINA GUINEA   guinea fowl

GALLINA PEPITORIA   chicken fricassee in saffron and garlic sauce

GANSO   goose

GANSO CON ACEITUNAS   roast goose stuffed with veal, ham, garlic, onion

GELATINA AVE   cold, poached chicken stuffed with meat, rolled, covered with gelatin

HIGADILLOS   chicken livers

HIGADILLOS GELE OPORTO   chicken livers in port flavored aspic

JARDINERA   with carrots, peas and mixed vegetables

JULIANNA   shredded vegetables

LANGOSTA, POLLO Y   chicken and lobster braised with onion and tomato, with paste of garlic, almonds, chestnuts, chicken liver

MADRILEÑA   with sausage, tomatoes and paprika
MENUDILLOS   giblets
MENUDILLOS DE GALLINA   chicken giblets; livers, hearts, gizzards, kidneys
MENUDILLOS DE POLLO   cold poultry
MOLE GUAJALOTE   turkey dish of Mexico, with garlic, tortillas, onion, tomatoes, chocolate
MOLE POBLANO   chicken with sauce of chili peppers and chocolate
OCA   goose
PAELLA VALENCIANA   rice, chicken, pimentos, shellfish and saffron
PARRILLA   grilled over an open fire
PARRILLADA INGLESA   mixed grill
PATO   duck
PATO ARROZ, CON   duck and rice
PATO HORNO, AL   roast duck
PATO NABOS, CON   braised duck with turnips, onions in brown wine sauce
PATO NARANJA, CON   roasted duck in brown sauce, orange and lemon juice
PATO PERES   duck with pears
PATO PIÑA, CON   roast duck in brown sauce with pineapple juice
PATO RELLENO TRUFADO   roast duck stuffed with truffles
PATO SALVAJE ROYAL   roast wild duck
PATO SEVILLANO BRASEADO   braised duck in olive oil, broth, sherry, tomatoes, sliced orange
PAVO   turkey
PAVO ASADO   roast turkey
PECHUGA   poultry breast
PECHUGA AVE, DE   chicken breast and wing
PECHUGA KIEV   chicken breast stuffed with butter, breaded and pan fried
PECHUGA NEVA   poached breast in gelatin
PECHUGA POLLO RELLENA, DE   chicken breast stuffed with ham, onion, wine

PECHUGA PORTUGUESA   braised breast in tomato, bacon, oil

PECHUGA VILLEROI   poached chicken, breaded and deep fried

PEPITORIA CON GALLINA   rice and chicken fricassee with stuffed partridge and quail, rabbit with garlic

PICHONCILLO   squab

PICHONES   squabs *or* pigeons

PICHONES ESTOFADOS   braised stuffed squabs

PIERNA   leg

PINTADA   guinea fowl

POLLASTRE   chicken

POLLITO   spring chicken

POLLO   chicken

POLLO AJILLO, CON   roasted chicken with garlic

POLLO AJO, CON   braised chicken in garlic, wine, oil, clove and nutmeg

POLLO, ALAS DE   chicken wings in a sauce

POLLO AMERICANO   chicken breaded and grilled then roasted with tomatoes, bacon, fried potatoes, with sauce of pan juices and lemon butter; or split broiler with breadcrumbs, roasted with tomatoes, French fried potatoes and herb butter

POLLO ASADO   roast chicken

POLLO ASADO A LA BORDELESA   chicken sauteed with shallots and wine

POLLO ASADO CON SALSA NARANJA   roast chicken with orange sauce

POLLO AST GLASEADO   spit roasted chicken with honey cumin glaze

POLLO, CACEROLA DE   casserole of braised chicken with mushrooms, carrots, bacon, peas, garlic and sherry

POLLO CASTELLANA, A LA   braised chicken in butter, pan juices and wine

POLLO CATALANA, A LA   braised chicken with eggplant, peppers, tomatoes, wine, oil

POLLO CHANFAINA   braised or stewed chicken

POLLO CHILINDRÓN   sauteed chicken with peppers, tomatoes and olives

POLLO CHILINDRÓN, CON   chicken with a tomato and pepper accompaniment

POLLO SEVILLANO, CHULETAS DE   braised chicken in tomato sauce with onions and carrots

POLLO COCOTTE   braised chicken in a casserole with butter, bacon, onions, potatoes and sherry

POLLO COCOTTE SUBAROFF   chicken stuffed with goose liver and truffles, cooked and served in sealed casserole with Madeira truffles and stock

POLLO, CRESTAS DE   cocks' crests, poached in cream sauce

POLLO ENDIABLADO   chicken basted with mustard, lemon juice, pepper flavored butter, breaded and roasted

POLLO ESCABECHE, EN   stewed marinated chicken

POLLO ESTRAGÓN   roasted chicken with vegetables and tarragon and brown tarragon sauce

POLLO FRÍO   chicken served cold

POLLO FRITO   fried chicken

POLLO FRITO GRANADINA   chicken fried in oil, garlic and wine

POLLO, GUISADO DE   stewed chicken in sauce of cinnamon, cloves, onion, wine, garlic and butter

POLLO HIGOS, CON   chicken baked with wine and figs

POLLO HORNO, AL   roast chicken with garlic and sherry

POLLO JAMONCITO, CON   boned chicken legs stuffed with mushrooms, breaded and fried

POLLO LANGOSTA, CON   chicken braised with onion, tomato, cinnamon and lobster with garlic, almonds, chestnuts, chicken liver and chocolate made into a paste

POLLO MENESTRE, CON   chicken and vegetable soup-stew

POLLO, MUSLOS DE   chicken thighs boned and stuffed with meat mixture, breaded and fried

POLLO PARRILLA, A LA   grilled chicken
POLLO PEPITORIA   chicken braised in white wine,
almonds and garlic
POLLO PIBIL   chicken simmered in fruit juices
POLLO PIÑONES   sauteed chicken with pine nuts, arti-
chokes, ham, wine
POLLO RELLENO   stuffed chicken
POLLO RELLENO PERIGOT   chicken stuffed with liver
on a slice of tongue and wine sauce
POLLO RIOJANA, CON   chicken braised with tomatoes,
pepper, red pepper, onion, wine
POLLO SALTEADO   sauteed chicken
POLLO SALTEADO GODARD   chicken sauteed with
elaborate garnishings
POLLO SAMFAINA   chicken sauteed in wine with pep-
pers, eggplant and tomatoes
POLLO SEVILLANA   chicken fricassee with pimentos,
onion, garlic, tomato, wine, brandy and olives
POLLO VASCO   chicken braised in wine, tomatoes,
peppers, mushrooms, ham, onion and garlic
POLLO VIENÉS   chicken breaded, pan fried in butter
with lemon juice
POLLO VINO TINTO, CON   chicken sauteed with sau-
sage, wine and brandy
POULARDA   large roasting chicken
RAGÚ   stew *or* fricassee
ROMANA   dipped in batter and fried
SALPICÓN DE AVE   chicken with mayonnaise
VALENCIANA   with rice, tomatoes and garlic
VIZCAÍNA   with green peppers, tomatoes, garlic

Rice and Pasta

ALMEJAS ARROZ   clams with rice
ARROCES   rice
ARROZ   rice

ARROZ ALICANTINO   saffron flavored rice with peppers, tomatoes, artichoke hearts and boiled fish

ARROZ AZAFRÁN   saffron rice

ARROZ BACALAO, CON   rice, codfish, onion, tomato, potato, fish broth, garlic

ARROZ BANDA   rice with fish, shellfish, garlic, tomatoes, wine

ARROZ BLANCO   boiled rice

ARROZ CALABACÍN   rice with zucchini, red pepper, tomato, garlic, green beans

ARROZ CALDERO MURCIANA   fish, dried red peppers, garlic, shrimp, squid, tomato, fish broth

ARROZ CATALANA   rice, rabbit, sausage, pork ribs, ham and pea pods

ARROZ CORDERO, CON   rice with lamb, chick-peas, tomato, bacon, sausage

ARROZ COSTA BRAVA   rice with chicken, lobster, bacon, tomatoes, garlic

ARROZ COSTEÑO   rice with oven-browned crust, chick-peas, sausages, chicken, garlic, eggs

ARROZ COSTRA ALICANTINO   rice with meatballs, chicken, sausage, chick-peas, pork cubes and eggs baked on top

ARROZ COSTRADO HUEVOS   crusted rice with chicken, ham, sausages, chick-peas, onion, eggs

ARROZ CUBANA   oven cooked rice with fried eggs

ARROZ ESCARLATA   rice with tomatoes and prawns

ARROZ ESPAÑOLA   rice with chicken liver, pork, tomatoes

ARROZ HORNO, AL   rice, chick-peas, onion, tomato, garlic, potato, sausage

ARROZ LANGOSTA, CON   rice with spiny lobster

ARROZ MARINERO   rice with shellfish

ARROZ MARISCOS, CON   rice with shellfish

ARROZ MEJILLONES Y ALMEJAS, CON   rice with mussels and clams

ARROZ MEJILLONES, CON   rice with mussels

ARROZ MIRAMAR rice, mussels, shrimp, olive oil, pork, ham, onion, squid, firm fish, tomato, artichoke hearts

ARROZ NEGRO rice with squid, onion, fish broth, tomato, chili pepper, wine

ARROZ PARRILLADO rice, meats, chicken and vegetables

ARROZ, PATO CON roast duck with sausage and ham flavored rice

ARROZ POLLITOS, CON rice with chicken, wine, tomato puree, onion, ham, grated cheese

ARROZ POLLO, CON rice prepared in broth with chicken

ARROZ PRIMAVERA rice with spring vegetables

ARROZ ROSEXAT saffron rice pilaf cooked in a broth, served browned with sausages and pork and bacon meatballs

ARROZ SANTANDERINO rice with salmon and milk

ARROZ VALENCIANO rice with vegetables, chicken, shellfish

CABELLO DE ÁNGEL fine noodles; angel's hair

CANELONES stuffed pasta covered with sauce, grated cheese, baked

CANELONES A LA REINA stuffing of chicken and mushrooms with white sauce

CANELONES ROSSINI stuffing of ham, bacon, chicken livers, onions and tomatoes, with white sauce

CAZUELA DE FIDEOS noodle dish with beans and cold spices

CHANFAINA SALMANTINA dish of rice, giblet, lamb sweetbread and pieces of chorizo

CROQUETAS PAELLA, EN fried balls of paella rice mixture

ESPAGUETIS spaghetti

FIDEO thin noodle

FIDEOS some form of pasta

FIDEOS DE CAZUELA noodles with spareribs, sausages, ham and bacon

FIDEOS GORDOS large noodles

GRATIN cooked vegetables or pasta, baked in a casserole with butter, bread crumbs and grated cheese

LASAÑA   a wide flat noodle

LASAÑA HORNO   lasagna with alternating layers of mozzarella, ricotta cheese, meat-tomato sauce, baked

LASAÑA VERDE   green lasagna made with spinach dough

MACARRONES   macaroni

MARISCOS FIDEUA   noodles with fish, shrimp, tomatoes, fish broth

MOROS CRISTIANOS   rice, black beans, ham, garlic, green peppers

ÑOQUIS PARISINA   flour dumplings with cheese sauce, oven browned

NOUILLES   fresh noodles

NOUILLES VERDES   green noodles made with cooked spinach in the raw dough

PAELLA   stew of pork, rice, chicken, clams, shrimp

PAELLA ALICANTINA   rice, chicken and rabbit stew

PAELLA ARAGONESA   stew of rabbit, pork, squid, tomato, onion, peas, bell pepper, garlic and saffron

PAELLA BARCELONESA   stew of rice, chicken, chicken liver, squid, fish, onion, tomatoes, garlic, green pepper, mussels, shrimp, olive oil, sausage, peas, saffron, artichokes

PAELLA CATALANA   stew of rice, sausages, pork, squid, tomatoes, peppers and peas

PAELLA CODORNICES Y SETAS, CON   stew of rice, rabbit, pork, quail, tomato, beans, onions, mushrooms, garlic, pork ribs

PAELLA HUERTANA MURCIA   stew of rice, green beans, peas, lima beans, tomato, artichoke hearts

PAELLA MARINERA   stew of rice with fish, shellfish and meat

PAELLA MARISCOS CON POLLO, DE   stew with seafood and chicken

PAELLA MARISCOS, DE   rice and shellfish stew

PAELLA MILANESA   rice in broth with sauteed onion, wine and saffron

PAELLA PARRILLADA   rice containing chicken, meat,
   sausage, fish, seafood, onions, garlic, tomato and peas
PAELLA VALENCIANA   rice, chicken, pimentos, shellfish
   and saffron
PASTA ITALIANA   spaghetti
PASTAS BAVARAS   spatzle, small dumplings made of dough
PEPITORIA CON GALLINA   rice and chicken fricassee
   with stuffed partridge and quail, rabbit with garlic
PIMIENTOS RELLENOS   peppers stuffed with rice
RAVIOLES   dough squares with meat or other stuffing,
   boiled, served with sauce and grated cheese
ROSEXAT   saffron rice pilaf cooked in a broth with sau-
   sages and pork and bacon meatballs, browned in oven
SEMOLA   semolina
SPAGETTIS   spaghetti
SPAGETTIS A LA BOLOÑESA   spaghetti with meat and
   vegetable sauce
SPAGETTIS A LA INGLESA   spaghetti with veal gravy,
   grated Parmesan cheese, baked
SPAGETTIS BILBAÍNA   cooked spaghetti with crabmeat
   in a tomato sauce with onion, garlic, broth and paprika
SPAGETTIS ITALIANOS   spaghetti with butter and
   grated cheeses
SPAGETTIS NAPOLITANOS   spaghetti with tomato
   sauce, garlic and onion sauteed in olive oil with grated
   cheese
TALLARINES   noodles
TALLARINES CATALANOS   noodles in sauce with pork
   spare ribs, sausage, onion, tomato, garlic, almonds
VERMICELLI   thin spaghetti

Salads

ACEITUNAS   olives
ACEITUNAS NEGRAS   black olives
ACEITUNAS VERDES   green olives
ACHICORIA   chicory

ADEREZO   dressing
ALIÑADAS NEGRAS   black olives
ALIÑADAS VERDES   green olives
ALIÑO   salad dressing with herbs and cheese
AMANIDA   salad
AMANIDA BACALLA   salt cod salad
AMANIDA FAVES   bean salad
AMANIDA LLENTIES   lentil salad
AMANIDA MONGETS   black-eyed pea and salt cod salad
APIOS   celery
BERRO   cress
ENDIBIAS   endive
ENDIBIAS BELGAS   Belgian endive, vegetable with long, crispy leaves
ENSALADA   salad; also see ENTREMESES
ENSALADA ALMORAINA   salad with escarole, tomato, cumin, olive oil and wine vinegar
ENSALADA ANGUILAS, DE   salad of baby eels in garlic, olive oil and vinegar
ENSALADA APIO BLANCO, DE   salad with celery
ENSALADA ARENQUE, DE   herring salad
ENSALADA ARROZ, DE   salad with rice, mushrooms, oil, vinegar, garlic, anchovy, mustard
ENSALADA AVE, DE   chicken salad
ENSALADA BERROS, DE   watercress salad
ENSALADA BLANCA   salad with white beans, onion, oil and vinegar
ENSALADA CORAZÓN DE PALMITO, DE   canned heart of palm salad
ENSALADA CATALANA   salad with lettuce, onions, bell peppers, tomato, tuna, codfish, ham, sausage, hard-boiled egg
ENSALADA CATALINA   summer salad of romaine or curly endive lettuce, tomatoes, sweet raw onion, green and red peppers, green and black olives
ENSALADA CHAMPIÑÓN   mushroom and ham salad
ENSALADA COLAS DE CANGREJO, DE   crayfish salad

ENSALADA COMÚN   green salad

ENSALADA CORRIENTE   salad with seasonal local ingredients

ENSALADA ENDIBIAS QUESO Y CABRALES, CON endive salad with blue cheese

ENSALADA ESCALIBADA   artichoke, eggplant, pepper and tomato salad

ENSALADA ESCAROLAS, DE   salad with slightly bitter green head lettuce

ENSALADA ESPARTEROS, DE   salad with tuna, egg, potato, onion, capers

ENSALADA FRUTAS, DE   fruit salad

ENSALADA ILUSTRADA   salad with combination of ingredients

ENSALADA ITALIANA   Italian salad

ENSALADA JUDÍAS VERDES A LA VINAGRETA, DE salad with green bean, onion, oil and vinegar

ENSALADA KOSH KERA   salad with fish, lobster, pimiento, olives, eggs, oil and vinegar

ENSALADA LANGOSTA, DE   spiny lobster salad

ENSALADA LEGUMBRES, DE   mixed vegetable salad

ENSALADA MADRILEÑA   salad with lettuce, tomatoes, hard-boiled eggs, olive oil, vinegar

ENSALADA MIXTA   mixed salad

ENSALADA MURCIANA   salad with romaine lettuce, green peppers, cucumbers, tomatoes, onion, oil, vinegar

ENSALADA NACIONAL   potato salad with peas, tuna, ham, pimento

ENSALADA NARANJA Y QUESO, CON   salad with oranges and cheese

ENSALADA NIÇOISSE   salad of cooked and raw vegetables, marinated in oil and vinegar, topped with eggs, anchovies, tuna on a bed of lettuce

ENSALADA NORMAL   green salad

ENSALADA PAÍS, DEL   salad of seasonal local ingredients

ENSALADA PALMERA, DE   canned palm heart salad

ENSALADA PATATA Y REMOLACHA, DE   potato and beet salad

ENSALADA PEPINO, DE   cucumber salad

ENSALADA PIPARRADA   cucumber tomato and pepper salad

ENSALADA POLLO, DE   chicken salad

ENSALADA PRIMAVERA   spring salad with vegetables

ENSALADA RAQUEL   salad of boiled potatoes, artichokes, asparagus, celery, truffles with mayonnaise dressing

ENSALADA REMOLACHA, DE   red beet salad

ENSALADA RUSA   salad of cooked vegetables in mayonnaise sauce

ENSALADA SAN ISIDRO   mixed salad of onion, lettuce and tuna

ENSALADA SEVILLANA   salad with curly endive, tarragon, pitted olives, oil and vinegar

ENSALADA SURTIDA   mixed salad

ENSALADA TOMATE Y HUEVO, DE   salad with tomato and egg wedges, onion and vinegar

ENSALADA TOMATES, DE   tomato salad

ENSALADA VALENCIANA   green pepper, lettuce and orange salad

ENSALADA VARIADA   mixed green salad

ENSALADA VERDURAS, DE   vegetable salad

ENSALADA WALDORF   apples, celery, walnut, mayonnaise salad

ENSALADA ZARINA   salad of cooked potatoes, carrots, turnips, topped with cold salmon, lettuce, tomatoes and hard boiled egg, mayonnaise sauce

ENSALADILLA   mixed vegetable salad

ENSALADILLA RUSA   cooked potato and vegetable salad covered with mayonnaise

ESCAROLA   endive

ESQUEIXADA   shredded salt cod salad

ESQUEIXADA LLUC CAVIAR   marinated hake salad with caviar

ESQUEIXADA POLLASTRE   shredded chicken salad
LECHUGA   lettuce
MAYONESA   mayonnaise
NOPALITO   cactus leaf with salad dressing
PALMITO   palm heart
PEPINILLO   pickle
PEPINILLOS EN VINAGRE   pickled cucumbers
PEPINO   cucumber
PEREJIL   parsley
PESCADITOS CON ESCABECHE A LA CATALANA
   fried small marinated fish with pepper and garlic
PESCADITOS CON ESCABECHE A LA ANDALUZA
   fried small marinated fish Andalusian style, with
   saffron, ginger and garlic
PICADILLA   creamy almond dressing
PIPIRRANA   salad of green pepper, onion, tomato and
   marinated fish
PLATO RÉGIMEN CRUDO, DE   salad plate
RÁBANO   radish
SALPICÓN DE MARISCOS   shrimp and lobster salad in
   tomato sauce
TREMPO   salad
UMA SALADA PORTUGUESA   mixed green salad
VINAGRETA   oil and vinegar salad dressing
XATO   peppery salad of curly endive with meats and sausages
ZANAHORIAS   carrots

Sauces and Butters

AJIACEITE   garlic mayonnaise
AJOLIO   garlic flavored mayonnaise dressing served with fish
ALI-PEBRE   garlic, olive oil and paprika sauce
ALI-OLI   garlic mayonnaise
ALIÑO   salad dressing with herbs and cheese
ALIOLI   garlic flavored mayonnaise
AMBAS SALSAS   two sauces of chef's choice
BECHAMELLE   creamy white sauce

BEIXAMEL   bechamel sauce

CHILINDRÓN   thick tomato sauce with ham, red bell peppers, oil and garlic

CHILINDRONES   sauce made with pepper, tomato and fried onion

CHIMICHURRI   hot parsley sauce

CHORÓN   tomato flavored Bearnaise sauce

FRUTA CON ALIOLI   garlic mayonnaise with fruit

HOLANDESA   Hollandaise sauce, made with lemon juice flavored egg yolks and butter

HUEVOS CON ALIOLI   garlic mayonnaise with eggs

MAÎTRE D'HÔTEL SALSA   butter creamed with lemon juice

MANTECA NEGRA   browned butter

MANTEQUILLA   butter

MANTEQUILLA FUNDIDA   melted butter

MAYONESA   mayonnaise

MOJO   dressing made with oil, vinegar, garlic, salt, spices; for color: paprika for red, piquant peppers for picon, coriander for green

MORNAY   creamy cheese sauce

MOUSSELINE (SALSA)   Hollandaise sauce with added whipped cream

PICADA   sauce containing garlic, parsley, toasted almonds and chopped pine seeds

PICADILLA   creamy almond dressing

PICANTE   peppery

ROMESCO   sauce of olive oil, red pepper, bread, garlic, almonds, cognac, vinegar

SALMOREJO SALSA   sauce of bread croutons, garlic, salt, olive oil, vinegar and water ground in a mortar and pestle

SALPICÓN   tomato pulp, garlic, onions, olive oil, herbs simmered into a tomato sauce

SALSA   sauce

SALSA ALBUFERA   mushroom flavored creamy sauce

SALSA BEARNESA   egg yolk-butter sauce with wine and vinegar, thick and creamy

SALSA BLANCA   white sauce

SALSA CARNE   gravy
SALSA COLORADA   red sauce of tomatoes, garlic, eggs, almonds, olive oil, vinegar, pepper
SALSA CON SAMFAINA   sauce of oil, lard, onion, green peppers, eggplant, zucchini, tomatoes
SALSA DE MOSTAZA   creamy mustard-butter sauce
SALSA ESPAÑOLA   brown sauce with wine
SALSA HOLANDESA   thick sauce with lemon juice, egg yolks and butter
SALSA MANZANA, DE   appl esauce
SALSA MAYONESA, DE   mayonnaise
SALSA MAYORDOMO, DE   butter and parsley sauce
SALSA PER CALCOTS   grilled green onion sauce
SALSA PICANTE   hot pepper sauce
SALSA ROBERT   mustard flavored meat sauce with onion and white wine
SALSA ROMANA   sauce of bacon or ham, egg and cream
SALSA ROMESCO   peppery sauce of tomato, hot chili pepper, garlic, hazelnuts, olive oil, wine vinegar
SALSA ROMESCU   red sauce of oil, vinegar, hot pepper, garlic, onion, pimento and tomato puree
SALSA TÁRTARA   tartar sauce
SALSA TOMATE, DE   tomato sauce
SALSA VERDE   green sauce
SOFREGIT   sauce base
SOFRITO   fried sauce made with garlic, onion, tomato and parsley
SOFRITO SALSA   sauce of olive oil, onion, garlic, parsley and tomato

Sausages and Pâtés

AGUJA   filled baked pastry
AMEIJOAS CATAPLANA   steamed clams, sausages, ham and tomatoes
BUÑUELITOS CHORIZO   fritters made with chopped sausage

BUTIFARRA   spicy sausage
BUTIFARRA Y JUDÍAS   broiled sausage with white beans
BUTIFARRA Y SETAS   baked sausages and mushrooms
CACHELOS   boiled diced potatoes, cabbage, garlic, bacon, chorizo sausage
CHALUPAS   spicy Mexican dish of sausage, chili, onions
CHORIZO   sausage of pork, pork fat, spices, herbs and paprika
CHORIZO CON SIDRA   sausage and apples in hard cider sauce
CHORIZO DE OLLA   fried sausage preserved in pork fat
CHORIZO HOJALDRADO   sausage slices baked in pastry
COCA   open face baked pie with vegetable or meat topping
EMBUCHADO   pork sausage
EMBUTIDO   spicy sausage
EMPANADA   meat or fish pie baked with onion and peppers
EMPANADA ASTURIANA   baked sausage pie
EMPANADA BERBERECHA   baked clam pie
EMPANADA BONITA   baked tuna pie
EMPANADA DE LOMO   baked pork pie
EMPANADA DE SARDINAS   baked sardine pie
EMPANADA GALLEGA   chicken filled pastry
EMPANADA HORNO, AL   pastry with minced meat filling
EMPANADILLAS   small fried stuffed pastry turnovers
EMPANADILLAS DE ATÚN   small fried tuna stuffed pastry turnovers
EMPANADILLAS DE CHORIZO   chorizo sausage pastries
EMPANADILLAS JAMÓN   ham pastries
EMPANIDILLAS VALENCIANAS   pastries stuffed with ham and tuna
FARINATOS   sausage which is fried and served with eggs
FUETE   sausage
GRANADINA   eggplant and ground ham loaf
LOMBARDA RELLENA   baked sausage stuffed red cabbage
LOMO RELLENO SALCHICHA   sausage wrapped in pork slices, sauteed with onion, garlic, wine
LONGANIZA   sausage

MORCILLA   mild blood sausage
PASTEL   baked puff pastry pie sometimes with sausage, ham, peppers and onion or a meat loaf
PASTEL CHOCLO   puff pastry with corn, chopped beef, chicken, raisins and olives
PASTEL MURCIANO   baked veal, ham, pepper, tomato pie
PASTEL PERDIZ   partridge pâté
PASTEL PUERROS Y GAMBAS, CON   shrimp and leek pâté
PEPITOS   sandwich rolls
PEPITOS DE TERNERA   veal sandwich rolls
PERRITOS CALIENTES   hot dogs
RIOJANA   fried chorizo sausage with grilled tomato
SALCHICHA   sausage
SALCHICHA BLANCA ASTURIANA   breakfast sausage
SALCHICHA CHABLIS, EN   sausage poached in Chablis wine
SALCHICHA FRANKFURT   hot dog
SALCHICHA FRITA   fried sausage
SALCHICHA HIGOS AGRI-DULCES, CON   sausage with sweet and sour figs
SALCHICHA LONGANIZA, CON   rosemary flavored breakfast sausage
SALCHICHA RELLENA CON REPOLLO   sausage fried in cabbage leaf
SALCHICHÓN   salami
SALCHICHÓN VICH   Catalonian sausage
SALMÓN HOJALDRADO   puff pastry with salmon filling
SOBRASADA   salami; *or* spread of sausage with fat added on toast
SOBRASADA CON MALLORCA   pimiento spiced sausage from Majorca
TERNERA EN AGUJA   veal in baked pastry
TERNERA PASTEL   veal pâté
TERRINA   meat or fish paste usually in pastry shell
TERRINA DE CONEJO   rabbit pâté
TERRINA DE PERDIZ   partridge and liver pâté

Seafood

ABADEJO   codfish

ACEDÍAS   flounder

ACEDÍAS FRITAS   flounder pan fried in oil

ADOBO   marinated

AJO ARRIERO   pieces of seafood or fish in a garlic sauce
of tomatoes, bell peppers, hot pepper and olive oil

AJOLIO   garlic flavored mayonnaise dressing served with
fish

ALLI-PEBRE D'ANGUILES   eel in garlic sauce

ALMEJAS   clams

ALMEJAS AL HORNO   baked stuffed clams

ALMEJAS ARROZ   clams with rice

ALMEJAS ENDIABLADAS   clams in a spicy tomato sauce

ALMEJAS MARINERAS   clams in hot pimento sauce

ALMEJAS ROMESCO   clams in tomato sauce with hot
pepper, chili pepper, vinegar and garlic

ALMENDRITAS   small squid

AMEIJOAS CATAPLANA   steamed clams, sausages, ham
and tomatoes

ANCAS DE RANA   frogs' legs

ANCAS DE RANA A LA PROVENZAL   frogs' legs
sauteed in olive oil, garlic and parsley

ANCAS DE RANA A LA VALENCIANA   marinated and
fried frogs' legs

ANCHOA   anchovy

ANCHOVA   anchovy

ANCHOVAS FRITAS   deep fried anchovies

ANGUILA   eel

ANGUILA AHUMADA   smoked eel

ANGULAS   baby eels

ANGULAS BILBAÍNA   eels sauteed in olive oil with red
pepper and garlic

ANGULAS PIL PIL   eels sauteed in olive oil with red
pepper and garlic

ANGULAS VASCA   eels sauteed in olive oil with red
   pepper and garlic
ARENQUE   herring
ARENQUE AHUMADO   kippered herring
ARENQUE ESCABECHE   pickled herring
ATÚN   tuna fish
ATÚN ESCABECHADO   pickled tuna fish
ATÚN GUIPUZCOANA   fresh tuna, pan fried in oil, wine
   and onions
ATÚN SEVILLANO   fresh tuna fried in butter, marinated
   and simmered in wine, vinegar, garlic, oil and olives
ATÚN VASCO   tuna steaks baked in tomato and wine
BACALAO   dried salt cod fish
BACALAO AJO ARRIERO, CON   pieces of codfish
   braised in oil with garlic, tomatoes, red peppers
BACALAO BATURRA   pieces of cod, cream, garlic and
   scrambled eggs
BACALAO CASERO   codfish in garlic-oil sauce
BACALAO GOMES SA   salt cod with potatoes and onions
BACALAO LLAUNA   codfish pan-fried with olive oil,
   garlic, tomatoes, red pepper, wine, then oven browned
BACALAO NAVARRA   cod braised in garlic sauce, onion,
   tomato, chili pepper, sliced potatoes, rice and saffron
BACALAO PASAS Y PIÑONES, CON   codfish with
   raisins and pine nuts
BACALAO PIL PIL   codfish simmered and served in hot
   garlic olive oil
BACALAO RIOJANO   cod, oven baked in a casserole
   with sauteed onions and garlic, red bell peppers
BACALAO SALSA VERDE, CON   codfish simmered and
   served in green sauce of parsley, garlic, vinegar-soaked
   bread and butter
BACALAO SAMFAINA   cod sauteed in tomato, onion,
   eggplant, peppers
BACALAO VIZCAÍNA   cod with green peppers, potatoes, tomato sauce
BARBO   river fish

BERBERECHO   small cockle

BESUGO   sea bream, like red snapper or porgy

BESUGO BILBAÍNO   fish dipped in egg, fried in deep fat

BESUGO DONOSTIARRO   charcoal grilled sea bream fish

BESUGO HORNO, AL   baked red snapper

BESUGO MADRILEÑO   baked porgy in wine tomato sauce

BESUGO PIÑONES, CON   porgy sauteed in wine and
    pine nut sauce

BESUGO RELLENO   baked porgy stuffed with egg, ham,
    onion, pimiento

BOGAVANTE   lobster with claws *or* large crayfish with
    pincers

BOGAVANTE AMERICANA   boiled pieces of lobster or
    crayfish with sauce of tomatoes, onions, white wine,
    paprika or mild red pepper, oven browned

BOGAVANTES   large clawed lobster similar to Maine
    lobster

BOLINAS DE BACALAO   codfish cakes

BONITO   striped tuna fish

BONITO MARINERO   tuna slices pan-fried in olive oil,
    with tomato sauce, garlic, onion

BOQUERONES   smelts, fish like a large anchovy

BOQUERONES EN VINAGRE   smelts marinated in garlic
    vinegar

BOQUERONES EN VINAGRE FRITOS   fish marinated in
    garlic vinegar and fried

BRANDADA BACALLA   salt cod puree

BRANDADA CARXOFE   salt cod puree with artichoke

BRANDADA DE BACALAO   paste of mashed codfish
    and boiled potatoes with olive oil and milk

BUEYES DE MAR   large crabs with pincers

CABALLA   fish like mackerel

CABALLA VINAGRETA   mackerel lightly broiled, then
    covered with wine vinegar, garlic onion sauce

CALAMARES   squid

CALAMARES A LA PARRILLA   squid basted with garlic
    flavored olive oil and grilled

CALAMARES CON JEREZ   squid casserole with dry sherry
CALAMARES RELLENOS   squid fried in oil and stuffed
with chopped ham
CALAMARES ROMANOS   squid slices fried in batter
CALAMARES SALTEJATS ALL JULIVERT   squid sauteed
with garlic
CALAMARES TINTOS   squid braised in its own ink
CALDERADA   seafood stew
CALDERETA ASTURIANA   mixed fish stew
CAMARÓN   shrimp
CANAILLAS   sea snail
CANGREJO   crab
CANGREJO DE MAR   sea crab with hard shell
CANGREJO DE RÍO   river crayfish
CANGREJOS EN JEREZ   hard shell crabs in dry sherry
CARABINEROS   prawn with red shell
CARACOL   snail
CARPA   carp
CASTAÑOLA   sea perch
CASTAÑOLA CATALANA   sea perch with onions,
tomatoes
CATALANA   with onions, parsley and tomatoes
CAZUELA DE GAMBAS   prawns simmered in sauce
CENTOLLO   giant crab, like stone crab
CENTOLLO A LA DONOSTIARRA   crab meat simmered
in sauce of tomato and cognac served hot in shell
CENTOLLO GALLEGO   crab boiled, served whole,
cracked, cold
CEVICHE   fish marinated in lemon and lime juice
CHANGURRO   crab meat with sherry and brandy
CHANGURRO VASCO   crab meat simmered in sauce of
tomato, cognac and served hot in shell
CHANQUETES   small whitebait fish or sardines, deep
fried
CHICHARRO   horse mackerel
CHIPERONES   squid
CHIPERONES TINTA   squid braised in their own ink

CHIRLAS   small clam
CHOPA   fish like sea bream
CHUPE   thick soup or stew, usually with fish
CHUPE DE MARISCOS   scallops with creamy sauce and cheese
CIGALAS   sea crayfish with claws, like Maine lobster
CIGALAS COCIDAS   boiled crayfish
CIVET LLAGOSTA   lobster stew
CÓCTEL DE GAMBAS   prawn cocktail
CÓCTEL DE MARISCOS   cocktail of various seafoods
COLAS DE CIGALA   crayfish tails
CONCHAS FINAS   medium size clams
CONGRÍO   sea eel, served in sauce of tomato, garlic and oil
COQUINAS   small clams
CORBINA   sea bass *or* perch
COREGONO LAGO DE CONSTANZA   felchen from Lake Constance
COSQUERA   fish sauteed in olive oil with garlic, braised with wine, clams, peas and asparagus
COTZE   mussel
CROQUETAS   meat, fish or vegetable croquettes
CROQUETES LLAGOSTA, DE   lobster croquettes
CRUSTACEOS   shellfish
CURANTO   seafood, vegetables and pig cooked in an earthen well
DENTON   flat fish similar to pompano
DENTON MALLORQUINA   fish deep fried with sauce of oil, garlic and sherry
DORADA   fish similar to bream
EMPERADOR   swordfish
ENCEBOLLADO DE PESCADO   grilled fish covered with chopped onions, oil and vinegar
ERIZO MAR   sea urchin
ESCABECHE SARDINAS   pickled sardines
ESCOCIA   codfish
ESCOMBRO   mackerel
ESPADÓN   swordfish

ESPADÓN AHUMADO   smoked swordfish

ESPASA   swordfish

ESQUILAS   prawns

ESTURIÓN   sturgeon

ESTURIÓN CATALANO   sturgeon braised in onion, garlic, olive oil

FILETE LENGUADO EMPANADA, DE   breaded filet of sole

FLAMENCA   with green peppers, onions, tomatoes, peas and sausage

FRITURA MIXTA   deep-fried meats, chicken, vegetables or fish

FRITURA MIXTA PESCADOS   deep fried mixture of fish

FRUTAS DE MAR   seafoods

GAMBA   shrimp

GAMBA GRANDE   prawn

GAMBAS   large shrimp

GAMBAS AJILLOS, CON   shrimp with garlic mayonnaise sauce

GAMBAS, CÓCTEL DE   shrimp cocktail with mayonnaise sauce

GAMBAS DE LA BAYANA   prawns from the bay

GAMBAS GARBARDINA, CON   fried shrimp in a beer batter coating

GAMBAS JEREZ, CON   shrimp in dry sherry sauce

GAMBAS MAYONESA, CON   shrimp cocktail

GAMBAS SALSA PIPARRADA, CON   shrimp with tomato and pepper sauce

GAMBAS SALSA VERDE, CON   shrimp in green sauce

GAMBAS VILLEROY   boiled shrimp in a white bechamel sauce

GAMBONES   large prawns

GUSANOS   sea snail

HOJALDRA   puff pastry used for dessert or with fillings of meat and fish

HUACHINANGO   red snapper

HUEVAS ALIÑADAS   seasoned fish roe

JARDINERA   with carrots, peas and mixed vegetables

JULIANNA   shredded vegetables

JUREL   kind of mackerel

KOKOTXAS   hake fish

LAMPREA   sea or fresh water fish that looks like an eel

LAMPREA BORDELESA   fresh water fish with leeks and wine

LANGOSTA   lobster

LANGOSTA AJO ARRIERO, CON   lobster, onion, garlic, wine, vinegar

LANGOSTA AMERICANA   boiled pieces of lobster with sauce of tomatoes, onions, white wine, paprika or mild red pepper, oven-browned

LANGOSTA CARDINAL   pieces of boiled lobster with truffle slices on mushrooms, with grated cheese, oven browned, with tomato wine sauce

LANGOSTA CATALANA   lobster braised in white wine, onion and fish broth, with almond paste

LANGOSTA COSTA BRAVA, DE   lobster tails, mushroom, ham, scallion, wine

LANGOSTA HERVIDA   boiled lobster

LANGOSTA NEWBURG   lobster sauteed in thick white sauce, cream and wine

LANGOSTA POBRE   poor man's lobster, made from white fish, garlic, carrots, olive oil

LANGOSTA POLLO, Y   chicken and lobster braised with onion and tomato, with paste of garlic, almonds, chestnuts, chicken liver

LANGOSTA THERMIDOR   lobster braised in sherry cream sauce, mustard flavored fish stock, with cheese and oven browned

LANGOSTINOS   shellfish similar to shrimp; also see GAMBAS

LANGOSTINOS CLAVO, CON   boiled large shrimp in wine, pepper, clove, peppercorn sauce

LANGOSTINOS GRAN MESÓN   prawns in garlic onion sauce

LANGOSTINOS PARRILLA, A LA   shrimp grilled on a
  steel plate, basted with olive oil
LENGUADO   sole, a flounder-like fish
LENGUADO ALBARINO   filet of sole in wine mushroom
  sauce
LENGUADO ALMENDRAS, CON   filet of sole fried in
  butter with sliced almonds and lemons
LENGUADO AURORA   poached filets with creamy
  sauce, tomato puree added
LENGUADO CAFÉ PARÍS, DE   filet of sole poached in
  stock with truffles, mushrooms, asparagus tips, prawns
  in creamy lobster sauce
LENGUADO CHAMPAGNE, EN   filet of sole poached in
  champagne
LENGUADO COLBERT, CON   filet of sole breaded, deep-
  fried, stuffed with lemon butter
LENGUADO DELICIAS   filets of sole, poached, covered
  with creamy sauce
LENGUADO DONOSTIARRA, CON   filets immersed in
  butter and bouillon under a tomato sauce
LENGUADO ERMITAÑO   filets stuffed with crumbs,
  eggs, herbs, shallots, braised, served with creamy sauce
LENGUADO ESCORIAL   filet of sole oven poached in
  fish stock, covered with pink wine sauce
LENGUADO, FILETES DE   filets of sole, flat sea fish
LENGUADO FRITO   fried filet of sole with vegetables
LENGUADO GOUGONS   strips of filets, floured and
  deep fried
LENGUADO INGLÉS   filet of sole coated with beaten egg
  and bread crumbs and deep fried
LENGUADO, LAZOS DE   strips of filets, deep fried
LENGUADO LIMÓN, CON   filet of flounder in lemon
  wine sauce
LENGUADO MARGUERITE   filet of sole poached in wine
  with white sauce
LENGUADO MARGUERY   filet of sole poached in fish
  stock and wine, with creamy wine sauce, oven browned

LENGUADO MAYONESA VERDE, CON   fish filet with green mayonnaise sauce

LENGUADO MEUNIERE   whole sole floured, fried in butter

LENGUADO MILANESA, A LA   fish filet egg coated, breaded with crumbs and grated Parmesan cheese, then fried

LENGUADO MOLINERA   filets fried in butter on butter fried sliced mushrooms

LENGUADO MUJER   fish filet poached in white wine on mushrooms, oven browned

LENGUADO MURAT   strips of fried sole mixed with diced potato and artichoke hearts

LENGUADO NARANJA, CON   filet garnished with orange

LENGUADO NORMANDA   filet poached in fish stock covered with mushrooms, mussels and shrimp, covered with creamy sauce and oven browned

LENGUADO ORLI   filets breaded, deep-fried, served with lemon slices

LENGUADO OTELLO   filets on baked potatoes, creamed chopped shrimp, browned with creamy cheese sauce

LENGUADO PIÑONES, CON   fish filet with pine nuts and beef sauce

LENGUADO POPIETAS, CON   poached filets with creamy sauce

LENGUADO RELLENO   stuffed sole

LENGUADO ROMANO   poached filets on macaroni with grated Parmesan, anchovies, covered with white sauce and oven browned

LENGUADO SALSA DE NUECES, CON   sole filets in nut sauce

LENGUADO TÍO PEPE   poached in stock and sherry, covered with creamy sauce

LLAGOSTA   spiny lobster

LLAGOSTIN   prawn

LLAMANTO   lobster

LLOBARRO   sea bass
LLOBARRO FORN   baked sea bass
LLUC   hake fish
LOBARRO   bass
LUBINA   sea bass
LUBINA ALBUFERA   bass baked in garlic almond sauce
LUBINA CORTA CON CALDO   bass poached in a vegetable bouillon
LUBINA HINOJO, CON   bass marinated in oil, lemon juice and fennel, then grilled
LUBINA NARANJA, CON   fish fried, served with orange sections and orange flavored sauce
LUBINA SALSA TÁRTARA, CON   bass poached with tartar sauce
LUBINA SANTURCE   bass lightly fried, then oven baked with vinegar and fried minced garlic
LUBINA SUPREME VERÓNICA   filets poached in fish stock with orange liqueur, covered with a sauce, oven browned
LUBINA VINO BLANCO, CON   bass poached in white wine
LUBRICANTE   lobster with claws
LUCIO   pike
MADRILEÑA   with sausage, tomatoes and paprika
MAGANOS   squid
MALLORQUINA   highly seasoned fish and shellfish
MAR   fish and seafood
MARINERA   with mussels, onions, tomatoes
MARISCADA   mixed seafood grill
MARISCADA MARINERA   baked clams, mussels and other shellfish
MARISCADA PLANCHA, A LA   shellfish grilled over charcoal
MARISCOS   shellfish
MARISCOS COSTA BRAVA   shellfish in spiced tomato sauce
MEJILLONES   mussels marinated in oil, vinegar, capers, onion

MEJILLONES AMERICANOS   poached mussels with tomato sauce, simmered in oven

MEJILLONES BERCY   poached mussels in white wine, served with sauce of reduced poaching liquor

MEJILLONES CON SALSA VERDE   mussels in wine, oil, onion, garlic sauce

MEJILLONES GRATINADOS   baked mussels and mushrooms

MEJILLONES MARINEROS   mussels simmered in white wine, served in this steaming liquor

MEJILLONES POULETTE   poached mussels on half-shell with creamy stock mushroom sauce

MEJILLONES RELLENOS   poached mussels on half-shell with garlic butter

MERLUZA   hake, like codfish

MERLUZA AMERICANA   hake breaded and pan fried in sauce of oil, wine, onions, cheese

MERLUZA ANZUELO, CON   hake fritters

MERLUZA BATELERA   hake poached with puree of mussels and cream

MERLUZA BILBAÍNA   hake dipped in egg, fried in deep fat

MERLUZA BLANCA   hake poached with sauce on the side or oil and vinegar

MERLUZA CATALANA   braised hake

MERLUZA, COLA DE   tail of hake

MERLUZA CON AJILLO   poached hake with garlic flavored mayonnaise

MERLUZA COSQUERA   hake lightly fried in olive oil with garlic, wine, sauteed clams

MERLUZA, EMPAREDADOS DE   fried hake and ham slices

MERLUZA CECILIA, FILETE DE   hake pan fried in butter with asparagus tips

MERLUZA GALLEGA   baked fish with potato, paprika, onion, clove

MERLUZA GRANADINA   hake with fried garlic, peppers, onions, tomatoes, wine, simmered in oven

MERLUZA HERVIDA   hake poached in sauce

MERLUZA HORNO, AL   baked hake with potatoes and tomato sauce

MERLUZA JAIZKIBEL   cod or hake in rich wine sauce

MERLUZA KOSKERA   hake sauteed with clams, olive oil, garlic, wine, asparagus and green peas

MERLUZA MADRILEÑA   codfish stuffed with ham, cheese, bread crumbs battered and fried

MERLUZA MARINERA   poached hake filets with tomato and almond sauce

MERLUZA PAPEL CON JAMÓN, EN   hake marinated with slices of ham, sealed in oiled paper and oven baked

MERLUZA PLANCHA, A LA   hake grilled on a steel plate

MERLUZA PRIMAVERA   poached filets with green cream sauce

MERLUZA, PUDÍN DE   pudding of mashed hake, onion, tomato paste, oil, cooked, chilled and covered with mayonnaise

MERLUZA REBOZADA   battered and deep-fried hake

MERLUZA RIOJANA   hake with a tomato puree, peppers and garlic olive oil

MERLUZA ROMANA   battered and deep-fried hake

MERLUZA ROMESCA   hake in peppery sauce

MERLUZA SALSA VERDE, CON   hake with garlic, clams, green peas, asparagus

MERLUZA SIDRA, CON   fish in cider with clams, onion, potatoes, garlic

MERLUZA TROPICAL   hake sauteed and baked with bananas, onion, raisins, almonds, pineapple and sherry

MERLUZA VASCA   slices of hake simmered in oil with garlic, then put in earthenware casserole with sauce of fish stock, garlic and parsley and simmered in oven

MERO   halibut, pollack or sea bass

MERO BILBAÍNA   baked halibut with peppers

MERO BORGOÑONA   halibut poached in red wine

MERO CANTÁBRICO   halibut poached with sauce from onions, garlic, potato, parsley, olive oil and vinegar
MERO HORNO, AL   baked halibut with potatoes and onion
MERO MARINERO   halibut fried in oil, simmered with onion, bell pepper and garlic
MERO PLANCHA, A LA   halibut grilled on a steel plate
MERO SALSA VERDE, CON   pollock in green sauce
MOLINERA   fish floured and pan fried in butter
MOLUSCO   snail, mussel, clam
MUJOL   mullet
MUJOL HUEVAS   mullet roe, pan fried in butter
MUSCO GRATINATS   gratineed mussel
NAVAJAS   razor fish
NECORAS   crab
OLLA PESCADOS   seafood stew
OSTIONES   small shellfish, like oysters
OSTRAS   oyster
OSTRAS, 1/2 DOCENA DE   half a dozen oysters
OSTRAS MORNAY   poached oysters with white cheese sauce and oven browned
PAELLA   stew of pork, rice, chicken, clams, shrimp
PAELLA MARISCOS, DE   rice and shellfish stew
PAELLA VALENCIANA   stew of rice, chicken, pimentos, shellfish and saffron
PARRILLA   grilled over an open fire
PARRILLADA INGLESA   mixed grill
PARRILLADA MARISCOS   broiled seafoods or fish
PATILLA   prawn sized lobster
PEIX   fish
PERCA   perch fish
PERCEBE   barnacle
PERCEBES   goose barnacles
PERICONA   stew containing cod, oil, dry peppers and garlic
PESC VI I SALVIA   fish with wine and sage
PESCADILLA   fresh haddock

PESCADITO FRITO   deep-fried fish

PESCADO   fish

PESCADO ARROZ, CON   fish and rice

PESCADO CLEOPATRA, A LA   fish boned and stuffed with creamed whiting paste, poached with white wine sauce

PESCADO FRITO GADITANA   fish fried in olive oil

PESCADO GUISADO   fish stew

PESCADO VERACRUZ   fish, Mexican style, with garlic and olives

PEZ ESPADA   swordfish

PEZ ESPADA DE BILBAÍNA   swordfish simmered with garlic, pepper and oil

PIXIN   angler fish

PLATIJA   flounder

PULPA CON PATATINES   stewed octopus with potato, onion, garlic

PULPITOS   small octopus

PULPO   octopus

PULPO GALLEGO   octopus boiled in a sauce of paprika, pepper, garlic, olive oil

PULPO VINAGRETA, A LA   octopus boiled and marinated in wine vinegar, served cold

QUENELLE   dumpling of pastry and fish paste with a creamy sauce

QUISQUILLA   very small shrimp

RABAS   fried squid

RANAS   frogs

RAPE   firm white fish

RAPE AMERICANO   fish braised in tomato sauce made from oil, wine, onions and tomatoes

RAPE ESTILO CADAQUES   fish braised with mussels, prawns in sauce

RAPE GRELOS Y ALMEJAS, CON   fish with collard greens and clams

RAPE GRENADINA, CON   oven baked fish with sauce of garlic, onion, peppers, tomatoes, wine and olive oil

RAPE JEREZ, CON   baked white fish in sherry sauce

RAPE ORLY   battered and deep-fried fish

RAPE RIOJANA, CON   fish braised in oil, onion, garlic, peppers and tomato sauce

RAPE ROMESCADA   fish braised in spicy tomato suace with oil, onion, red wine, garlic

RAVAS   bits of fried octopus

RAYA   skate, sea ray

REGAÑAOS   pastry with sardines and red pepper in the crust

REO   trout

RÓBALO   haddock fish

RODABALLO   turbot, flounder- like fish

RODABALLO ARLESIANA   turbot braised in wine stock with sauce from butter, flour and fish stock, oven-browned

RODABALLO CON SALSA ALBUFERA   turbot poached with mushroom cream sauce with bell peppers

ROLLO DE MERLUZA   fish steak fried with ham and eggs in green sauce

RUBIO   red mullet

SÁBALO   shad

SALMÓN   salmon, fish

SALMÓN AHUMADO   smoked salmon

SALMÓN RIN   Rhine salmon

SALMONETES   red mullets

SALMONETES ANDALUCES   mullets lightly battered and deep fried

SALMONETES BERCY   mullets grilled with a white wine sauce

SALMONETES FRANCILLÓN   mullets broiled on toast

SALMONETES GRENOBLESES   mullets pan fried with browned butter, capers and lemon

SALMONETES MIRABEAU   mullets fried in anchovy butter

SALMONETES PARRILLA, A LA   mullets grilled with lemon

SALPICÓN DE MARISCOS   shrimp and lobster salad in tomato sauce

SANCOCHO   sama (regional fresh fish) and boiled
   potatoes
SARDINAS   sardines
SARDINAS ENSARTADAS   skewered sardines
SARDINAS MONTAÑESAS   sardines boiled in grape
   leaves with onion, tomato, garlic, wine, mint
SENTOLLA   large crab
SEPIA   cuttlefish
SHANGURRO   stuffed crab
SOLLA   plaice *or* flounder
SUQUILLO DE PESCADORES   fish soup-stew
TALLINA   clam *or* mussel stew
TALLINA CATALANA   clams in tomato garlic sauce
TENCA   tench, fresh water fish
TOMATES RELLENOS RIA AROSA   tomatoes stuffed
   with shrimp, clams, onions, wine, cognac
TONYINA   tuna
TORTILLITAS CON CAMARONES   shrimp pancakes
TORTUGA   turtle
TRUCHA   trout
TRUCHA ALMENDRAS, CON   trout fried in butter with
   sliced almonds and browned butter
TRUCHA ASTURIANA   pan fried trout with bacon and
   tomato, paprika, lemon sauce
TRUCHA CREMA, CON   trout oven simmered in shallot,
   garlic, wine and cream sauce
TRUCHA ESCABECHADA   marinated trout, served cold
TRUCHA FILIPE V   fried trout and bacon, on milk soaked
   bread, covered with orange slices on cooked cabbage
   and oven baked
TRUCHA FRITA ASTURIANA   trout fried in butter
TRUCHA NAVARRA   pan fried trout stuffed with ham
TRUCHA, SARTÉN DE   trout sauteed in butter and oil
TRUCHA SEGOVIANA   trout fried in olive oil, with
   sauce of garlic, ham and lemon
TRUCHA WHISKEY   pan fried trout in butter, flamed
   with whiskey

TURBO   turbot
URTA   sea bass fish *or* porgy
URTA ROTENA   baked porgy and peppers with brandy
URTA SAL   porgy baked in salt accompanied with sauce
VALENCIANA   with rice, tomatoes and garlic
VEIRAS GRATINADAS   baked scallops in wine
VENERA   scallop
VENTRESCA ACEITE   belly meat of tuna in olive oil
VIEIRAS   scallops in the shell, with pepper, onions,
   parsley and bread crumbs, put into the oven
VIEIRAS GALLEGAS   scallops braised in onion sauce
   with garlic, peppers and wine
VIEIRAS SAN JACOBO   scallops on the half-shell, in a
   thick tomato sauce, served oven-browned
VIEIRAS SANTIAGO   baked scallops with brandy and
   wine in shells
VIVAS   raw oysters on the half shell
VIZCAÍNA   with green peppers, tomatoes, garlic
ZAMBURIÑA   a scallop
ZARZUELA   seafood chowder *or* stew
ZARZUELA DE PESCADO   fish with seasoned sauce

Soups

AJIACO BOGOTANO   chicken soup with potatoes
AJO BLANCO   gazpacho made with oil, almonds and
   garlic, cold water, a few grapes
AJO BLANCO CON UVAS   cold soup of almonds, garlic,
   vinegar soaked bread, white grapes
BISQUE   creamy soup of pureed seafood
BISQUE CON CANGREJOS   pureed seafood with crab
BISQUE CON LANGOSTA   pureed seafood with spiny lobster
BISQUE CON LANGOSTINOS   pureed seafood with
   large prawns
BISQUE HOMARD   pureed seafood with lobster
BORTSCH POLONESA   Polish red beet soup with other
   vegetables and sausages

BULLABESA   fish soup stew
BULLABESA MARSELLA   soup with fish and shellfish, garlic, onions, tomatoes
CALDERETA DE CODORNICES   quail and onions potted in chicken broth
CALDERETA DE LANGOSTA   lobster, onions, garlic, tomatoes in fish broth
CALDILLO DE CONGRÍO   conger-eel soup with tomatoes and potatoes
CALDO   meats or fish, vegetables, soup bones made into a broth
CALDO COCIDO   liquid part of soup-stew
CALDO COLADO   liquid part of soup-stew
CALDO DE CARNE   beef broth
CALDO DE GALLINA   chicken soup
CALDO DE PERRO GADITANO   fish broth, onion, garlic, lime juice and orange juice
CALDO DE PESCADO   fish broth
CALDO DE POLLO   chicken soup
CALDO GALLEGO   thick soup stew of cabbage, potatoes, beans, ham, sausage, spare ribs
CALDO GALLEGO BURGUÉS   smoked ham and bacon, veal, sausage, chicken, white beans, cabbage, turnips
CALDO GALLEGO CAMPESINO   soup of white beans, smoked ham and bacon, onion, cabbage, turnips
CALDO PARTERO   soup of various meats and vegetables
CALDO VERDE   potato and kale soup with sausage
CALLOS GALLEGOS   soup of tripe, chick-peas, sausage, onion, garlic, wine
CANJA   chicken soup with lemon and mint
COCIDO ANDALUZ   beef, pork, sausage, squash, green beans, garlic cooked into a soup-stew
COCIDO MADRILEÑO   a soup-stew of chick-peas, veal or beef, ham, salt pork, potatoes, sausage, cabbage, chicken, carrots, onions, pig's foot and garlic
CONSOMÉ   clear broth of meat, chicken or other stock
CONSOMÉ AVE, DE   chicken and vegetable soup

CONSOMÉ COLBERT   consommé garnished with vegetables and poached egg

CONSOMÉ CRECI   consommé with pureed carrots and rice

CONSOMÉ DE POLLO   chicken and vegetable soup

CONSOMÉ DOBLE   double strength consommé

CONSOMÉ EUGENIA MONTIJO   consommé with truffle and slices of chicken breast poured over egg yolk

CONSOMÉ FIDEOS, DE   consommé with thin spaghetti

CONSOMÉ GELATINOSO   jellied consommé

CONSOMÉ GIRONDINE   beef consommé with ham and carrot strips

CONSOMÉ JEREZ, CON   chicken broth with sherry

CONSOMÉ JULIENNE   consommé with thin strips of cooked vegetables

CONSOMÉ MADRILEÑA, A LA   consommé with tomato pulp

CONSOMÉ MANZANA, DE   apple consommé

CONSOMÉ MOSCOVITA   cold consommé with caviar and whipped cream

CONSOMÉ NATURAL   plain consommé

CONSOMÉ PARMESANO   consommé with Parmesan cheese

CONSOMÉ PROFITEROLES, CON   consommé with filled or unfilled pastry shells

CONSOMÉ SIMPLE   plain broth

CONSOMÉ SOLERA   consommé with sherry

CONSOMÉ TAZA, EN   consommé in a cup

CONSOMÉ TRES FILETES, CON   consommé with tongue, chicken and truffles

CONSOMÉ YEMA, CON   consommé with beaten egg yolks and flour, minced chicken

CORDERO MENESTRA   lamb and vegetable soup-stew

CREMA   creamed soup with pureed vegetables, seafood, meat, chicken or fish

CREMA AVE, DE   cream of chicken soup

CREMA CARDENAL, DE   lobster soup with added cream

CREMA CAROLINA   cream of chicken soup with cream and cooked rice added

CREMA CARRAMARES, DE   crab bisque with shrimp, onion, carrots, leek, tomato
CREMA CHAMPINOÑES, DE   cream of mushroom soup
CREMA CULTIVADORA   vegetable soup with bacon
CREMA DE POLLO   cream of chicken soup
CREMA ESPÁRRAGOS, DE   cream of asparagus soup
CREMA ESPINACAS, DE   cream of spinach soup
CREMA FAVES, DE   cream of bean soup
CREMA GALLINA, DE   cream of chicken soup
CREMA GUISANTES, DE   cream of pea soup
CREMA LADY CURZÓN   turtle soup with curry powder and whipped cream
CREMA LANGOSTA, DE   cream of spiny lobster soup
CREMA LEGUMBRES, DE   cream of vegetable soup
CREMA MARISCOS, DE   cream of seafood soup
CREMA PRINCESA   cream soup with pieces of chicken breast and asparagus
CREMA REINA   cream of chicken soup
CREMA SOLERA   cream soup with sherry
CREMA SOLFERINO   pureed tomato and potato soup
CREMA ST. GERMÁN   cream of pea soup
CREMA TOMATE, DE   cream of tomato soup
CREMA PERDIZ   cream of partridge soup
ESCUDELLA   soup *or* stew
ESCUDELLA DE PAJES   peasant soup stew
ESCUDELLA PAYES   soup-stew of meats, sausage, cabbage, garbanzo beans, potatoes, vegetables
FABADA CON ALMEJAS   soup of white beans, onion, garlic, chili pepper, carrots, wine, clams
GAZPACHO   iced tomato and cucumber soup
GAZPACHO AJO BLANCO, CON   iced soup with almonds, garlic, oil, vinegar, grapes
GAZPACHO ANDALUZ   iced soup with tomatoes, green peppers, garlic, olive oil, wine vinegar, bread, ice water
GAZPACHO EXTREMEÑO   iced soup with garlic, green pepper, bread, eggs, olive oil, wine vinegar, ice water

GAZPACHO MADRILEÑO   iced soup with green peppers, tomatoes, garlic, olive oil, ice water, cucumber, bread cubes, wine vinegar, cumin seed

GAZPACHO MALAGÁN   iced soup with almonds, bread, wine vinegar, garlic, ice water, olive oil, white grapes

GAZPACHO SEVILLANO   iced soup with garlic, green pepper, onion, tomatoes, cucumber, olive oil, wine vinegar, ice water

GAZPACHUELO   fish soup with halibut, wine, clam juice, potatoes, vinegar

GRATINADA CEBOLLA   onion soup with croutons and cheese

HUEVO ESCALFADO   soup with poached egg

LACÓN GRELOS   boiled pork hocks, potatoes, sausage, Swiss chard

LOCRO   corn soup stew of South America

MARMITKO   soup of tuna, tomato, onion, brandy, potatoes, green pepper

MENESTRA   green vegetable soup

MENESTRA POLLO, CON   chicken vegetable soup

MENESTRONE   vegetable soup

MOJE MANCHEGO   cold broth with black olives

OLAIGUA   olive oil soup

OLIAIGUA TOMATES   olive oil soup with tomatoes

OLLA   stew *or* soup

OLLA DE ESCUDELLA CON CARNE   soup with boiled meats and vegetables

PASTITAS   soup dumplings

PELOTA   fried meat dumplings

PEQUEÑA MARMITA   soup stew

POLLO MENESTRE, CON   chicken and vegetable soup-stew

POTAJE   soup; also see SOPAS

POTAJE ANDALUZ   garbanzo bean soup

POTAJE ESPINACAS Y GARBANZOS, CON   spinach, onion, chick-peas, garlic, ham

POTAJE GARBANZOS, CON   soup with garbanzo beans
POTAJE JUDÍAS BLANCAS O VERDES, CON   soup with
   white or green beans
POTAJE MORCILLA Y TOCINO, CON   sausage and
   bacon soup
POTAJE VIGILIA, DE   soup with garbanzo beans, fish,
   spinach, onions, garlic, almonds, egg yolk
POTE   meat and vegetable soup-stew
POTE ASTURIANO   soup stew with cabbage, pig's foot,
   sausages, bacon, ham and white beans
POTE GALLEGO   soup stew with pork shoulder, white
   beans, potatoes, sausages, tomatoes, turnip greens, veal
   and chicken
PUCHERO   beef soup with vegetables
PURÉ GUISANTES, DE   split pea soup
PURÉ LAMBALLE   puree of pea soup and tapioca
PURÉ LEGUMBRES, DE   pureed mixed vegetable soup
PURÉ LENTEJAS, DE   pureed lentil soup with bacon and
   onions
PURÉ PARMENTIER   pureed potato soup
PURÉ SOLFERINO   pureed soup of tomato and potato
PURRUSALDA   dried salt codfish, leeks, potatoes, garlic
   made into a soup-stew
SOPA   soup; also see CREMAS, CONSOMES
SOPA AJO Y HUEVO, DE   garlic soup with egg
SOPA AJO Y PESCADO, DE   garlic soup with fish stock
SOPA AJO, DE   garlic soup with eggs
SOPA ALBÓNDIGAS, DE   meatballs of veal and chicken
   in chicken broth
SOPA ALENTEJANA   coriander and garlic soup with
   poached eggs
SOPA ANCAS DE RANA, DE   frog's legs soup
SOPA ARROZ, DE   rice cooked in bouillon with chicken
   livers, vegetables or meats
SOPA BOLETS, DE   mushroom soup
SOPA CANTÁBRICA   fish soup

SOPA CASTELLANA   bread, preferably the broth of a stew, ham, sometimes a poached egg and garlic

SOPA CEBOLLA, DE   onion soup

SOPA CLARA   clear soup

SOPA COCIDA   soup part of soup-stew, with rice or pasta

SOPA CODA BUEY, DE   oxtail soup

SOPA COLA DE BUEY, DE   oxtail soup

SOPA CREMA, DE   cream of chicken

SOPA CUARTO DE HORA, DE   soup with olive oil, ham, shrimp, peas, tomatoes, onion, clams, boiled egg, rice

SOPA DE ALMENDRAS Y CEBOLLA   onion and almond soup

SOPA DEL DÍA   soup of the day

SOPA ESPAÑOLA   spiced soup with rice, tomatoes and peppers

SOPA ESPESA   thick soup

SOPA FIDEOS, DE   soup with noodles or pasta

SOPA FREDOLICS   wild mushroom soup

SOPA GALLINA CON PASTA, DE   chicken noodle soup

SOPA GARBANZOS Y CHORIZO, DE   chick-peas, sausage, garlic, pepper and bacon soup

SOPA GUISANTES, DE   pea soup

SOPA IMPERIAL   chicken and veal broth thickened with tapioca, with sherry and cubes of wine-flavored custard; cream of rice and tapioca soup; consommé with egg yolks and ham

SOPA JAMÓN, CON   soup with ham

SOPA JULIANA   vegetable soup with garlic

SOPA LANGOSTA, DE   spiny lobster soup

SOPA LEGUMBRES, DE   vegetable soup

SOPA LENTEJAS, DE   lentil soup

SOPA MALAGUEÑA   seafood soup with saffron, absinthe liquor, egg yolks, croutons

SOPA MARINERA   seafood soup

SOPA MARISCOS, DE   seafood soup

SOPA MARISQUERA   seafood soup

SOPA MEJILLONES, DE   mussel soup

SOPA MENUDO, DE   chicken giblet soup

SOPA MERLUZA, DE   hake fish soup

SOPA MOSCOVITA   milk and egg based soup with nutmeg seasoning

SOPA PANELA, DE   garlic soup with chick-peas, mint and croutons

SOPA PASTA, DE   soup with pasta

SOPA PATATAS, DE   potato soup

SOPA PAVESA   beef broth poured over toasted bread topped with raw egg and grated cheese, then browned

SOPA PESCADO CATALÁN, DE   fish soup with shellfish, fish, onion, tomato, olive oil, garlic

SOPA PESCADO GADITANA, DE   fish soup with garlic, onion, orange juice

SOPA PESCADO VASCA   fish soup with mussels, carrots, onion, shallots, olive oil, cognac, butter

SOPA PESCADO, DE   fish soup

SOPA PESCADORES   fish soup

SOPA PICADILLO, DE   thick soup with chicken, veal or ham, with beaten egg poured into hot soup before serving

SOPA PICANTE   goulash soup

SOPA PUCHERO, DE   beef soup

SOPA QUESO, DE   soup with cheese

SOPA RABO DE BUEY, DE   oxtail soup with vegetables and wine

SOPA RAPE, DE   fish soup with onions, garlic, tomato, celery, bread, vinegar, nuts and spices

SOPA REAL   clear broth with pastries or dumplings

SOPA SEVILLANA   highly seasoned fish soup

SOPA TOMATE, DE   tomato soup

SOPA TORTUGA, DE   turtle-rice soup

SOPA TRUCHA, DE   trout soup

SOPA TURBOT Y GAMBAS, DE   fish and prawn soup

SOPA VERDURAS, DE   vegetable soup

SOPA VIGILIA, DE   shellfish and fish soup with vegetables, sherry and hard-boiled egg

SUQUET   fish stew-soup of clams, mussels, garlic,
   almonds, fish broth
SUQUILLO DE PESCADORES   fish soup-stew
TAZA   soup served in a cup
VICHYSSOISE   chilled, creamed leek and potato soup

Spices, Condiments, and Herbs

ACEITE   oil
AJO   garlic
ALBAHACA   basil
ALIOLI   garlic flavored mayonnaise
AZAFRÁN   saffron
CANELA   cinnamon
CONDIMENTO   relish
ENELDO   dill
ESPECIE   spice
ESTRAGÓN   tarragon
GITANILLA   with garlic
HIERBA   herb
HIERBAS FINAS   chopped mixture of herbs
JENGIBRE   ginger
LAUREL   bay leaf
MEJORANA   marjoram
MELAZA   molasses
MENTA   mint
MOSTAZA   mustard
NUEZ MOSCADA   nutmeg
PEREJIL   parsley
PERIFOLLO   chervil
PICANTE   peppery
PIMENTÓN   paprika
RÁBANO PICANTE   horse radish
ROMERO   rosemary
SAL   salt
SALVIA   sage
TOMILLO   thyme

VAINILLA   vanilla
VINAGRE   vinegar

Tortillas

ENCHILADA   Mexican stuffed cornmeal pancake
ENCHILADA ROJA   cornmeal pancake filled with
   sausage dipped in red sweet pepper sauce
ENCHILADA VERDE   cornmeal pancake stuffed with
   poultry or meat and braised in a green tomato sauce
TACO   cornmeal or wheat pancake with meat or chicken
   filling, served with a spicy sauce
TAMAL   pastry dough with meat or fruit filling, steamed
   in corn husks
TAMALES   ground meat rolled in cornmeal dough
TAMALES CALIENTES   hot tamales
TORTILLA   omelette plain or with cheese, ham, mush-
   rooms, chicken livers, seafood filling; also see HUEVOS
TORTILLA ABUELO   omelette with parsley and fried
   bread cubes
TORTILLA AJITOS SILVESTRES, CON   omelette with
   young, wild garlic
TORTILLA ALICANTINA   omelette with onion, shrimp,
   asparagus, ham and tomato
TORTILLA AMPURDANESA   omelette with cooked
   white beans
TORTILLA ANDALUZA   omelette with sauteed
   tomatoes, ham, pimiento, mushrooms
TORTILLA ANGUILAS, CON   omelette with fried baby
   eels
TORTILLA ARANJUEZ   omelette with asparagus tips
TORTILLA ASTURIANA   omelette with tuna fish, onion
   and tomato
TORTILLA ATÚN ESCABECHADO, DE   omelette with
   marinated tuna fish and onion
TORTILLA ATÚN, DE   omelette with potatoes, spinach,
   chunks of tuna

TORTILLA BACALAO, DE   omelette with codfish and
  onion
TORTILLA BETANZOS   potato omelette
TORTILLA BUENA MUJER   fried bacon, fried onion and
  mushroom omelette
TORTILLA CATALANA   omelette with sauteed tomatoes,
  green pepper and eggplant
TORTILLA CHAMPIÑONES, CON   omelette with mush-
  room, ham, garlic
TORTILLA CHANGET   omelette with fried whitebait fish
TORTILLA CHORIZO, CON   omelette with spicy sausage
TORTILLA COMBINADA   omelette with combination of
  local ingredients
TORTILLA CONFITURA, CON   jam omelette
TORTILLA CORUÑESA   omelette with potatoes and
  cured ham
TORTILLA DÁTILES, CON   omelette with shrimp, ham,
  dates, tomato sauce
TORTILLA DE GRANADA   omelette made with lamb
  sweetbreads, chicken liver and kidney with white wine
TORTILLA DE SU ELECCIÓN   omelette of your choice
TORTILLA DULCE   jam omelette
TORTILLA ESCABECHE, CON   omelette with pickled fish
TORTILLA ESPAÑOLA   omelette with sliced potatoes
  and onions fried in oil
TORTILLA ESTRAGÓN, CON   omelette with tarragon
TORTILLA EXTREMEÑA   omelette with sausage and
  potatoes
TORTILLA FINES DE HIERBAS, CON   omelette with
  chopped fresh herbs
TORTILLA FRANCESA   plain tortilla
TORTILLA GALLEGA   omelette with potatoes, ham, red
  sweet peppers and peas
TORTILLA GAMBAS, CON   omelette with prawns and
  prawn sauce
TORTILLA GARBANZOS, CON   omelette with chick-peas
TORTILLA HABAS, CON   omelette with lima beans

TORTILLA HÚNGARA   omelette with onions sauteed
with ham and paprika cream sauce
TORTILLA JAMÓN, DE   ham omelette
TORTILLA JARDINERA   omelette with mixed vegetables
TORTILLA LACÓN, CON   omelette with pork shoulder meat
TORTILLA LEGUMBRES, CON   omelette with mixed,
diced, cooked vegetables
TORTILLA LORRENA   omelette with grilled bacon,
Gruyere cheese, cream and chives mixed in eggs
TORTILLA LYONESA   omelette with sliced fried onions
and eggs
TORTILLA MAGRA   lean ham omelette
TORTILLA MARINESCA   seafood omelette
TORTILLA MURCIANA   omelette with sauteed tomatoes,
onions, squash, eggplant
TORTILLA NAVARRA   omelette with tomatoes sauteed
with garlic, eggs on top, with fried sausage, cheese,
oven-baked
TORTILLA PAISANA   omelette with ham and vegetables
TORTILLA PATATA ESPAÑOLA, DE   Spanish potato omelette
TORTILLA PATATAS, DE   omelette made with potatoes
and onions, fried in olive oil
TORTILLA SABOYARDA   omelette of eggs mixed with
Swiss cheese and poured over sauteed potatoes
TORTILLA SACROMONTE   omelette made with fried
and breaded brain, lamb or veal testicles, potatoes, red
pepper and peas
TORTILLA SESOS, CON   omelette with sauteed brains
TORTILLA SETAS, CON   omelette with wild mushrooms
TORTILLITAS CON CAMARONES   shrimp pancakes

Vegetables

ACEDERA   sorrel
ACELGAS   Swiss chard
ACELGAS SALTEADAS MIGAS   Swiss chard sauteed
with croutons

AJILLO   young garlic

AJO   garlic

ALCACHOFAS   artichokes

ALCACHOFAS ANDALUZAS   artichokes fried with
chopped ham

ALCACHOFAS BORDALESAS   artichokes stewed in
butter with sliced potatoes

ALCACHOFAS POLONESAS   artichokes filled with
chopped egg and crumbs browned in butter

ALCACHOFAS SALTEADAS CON JAMÓN   quartered
artichokes with diced ham

ALCACHOFAS SERRANO   artichoke quarters with
Serrano ham

ALCAPARRA   caper

ALL   garlic

ALUBIA   bean

ALUBIAS   small lima beans

ALUBIAS BLANCAS   white lima beans

ALUBIAS ROJAS   red lima beans

ALUBIAS VERDES   green lima beans

ALVERJINES   eggplants

ALVERJINES FARCIDES ANXOVE   stuffed eggplants
with anchovy

APIOS   celery

APIOS BRASEADOS CON TOCINO   braised celery with
bacon

APIOS MILANESA   celery heart casserole with butter and
grated cheese, oven browned

ARVEJAS PARTIDAS   split peas

ASADILLO   peppers roasted with garlic, tomato and oil

BAJOCA FARCIDES   peppers stuffed with rice, pork,
tomatoes and spices

BERENJENA   eggplant

BERENJENA CON QUESO   eggplant baked with a cheese
cover

BERENJENA FRITA   eggplant pan fried in oil

BERENJENA PARRILLADA   sliced and grilled eggplant

BERENJENA PROVENZAL   fried eggplant stuffed with
   tomato, garlic, onions, sprinkled with grated cheese and
   baked
BERRAZA   parsnip
BERZA   cabbage
BLEDOS   Swiss chard
BLEDOS PANSES PIÑONES   Swiss chard with raisins
   and pine nuts
BOLETA GRAELLA   grilled wild mushroom
BRÉCOL   broccoli
BRÓCULI   broccoli
CALABACÍN   zucchini *or* squash
CALABACÍN AL HORNO   baked zucchini
CALABACÍN RELLENO   zucchini stuffed with meat or
   other type of stuffing
CALABAZA   pumpkin *or* squash blossoms
CALCOT FRITAS   deep fried green onion
CALCOTADA   grilled green onions, spicy sauce
CANTARELA   mushroom
CARBONADA CRIOLLA   pumpkin stuffed with beef and
   baked
CARDO   cardoon, plant resembling artichoke
CAZOLADA   potato and vegetable stew with bacon and ribs
CAZUELA ARAGONESA   white beans with sausage
CEBOLLAS   onions
CEBOLLETA   chive
CEBOLLITAS   small onions
CEBOLLITAS RELLENAS   small stuffed onions
CHALOTE   shallot
CHAMPIÑONES   mushrooms
CHAMPIÑONES AJILLO   mushrooms stir-fried in olive
   oil with garlic chili pepper
CHAMPIÑONES BORDALESA, A LA   mushrooms
   sauteed in oil with onion, garlic, lemon juice
CHAMPIÑONES JEREZ, EN   mushrooms sauteed in
   sherry wine

CHAMPIÑONES SALTEADOS   mushrooms sauteed in garlic butter

CHAMPIÑONES SEGOVIANA   mushrooms sauteed in wine, garlic and bacon

CHAYOTE   Mexican squash

CHILE   chili pepper

CHILE NOGADO   green peppers stuffed with whipped cream and nut sauce

CHILE Y QUESO   spicy chilis and cheese

CHIRIVÍA   parsnip

CHUCRUT   sauerkraut

CIURENY   wild mushrooms

COL   cabbage

COL DE BRUSELAS   Brussels sprouts

COL DE BRUSELAS SALTEADO   sauteed Brussels sprouts

COL FERMENTADA   sauerkraut

COLIFLOR   cauliflower

COLIFLOR CON AJO ARRIERO   deep-fried cauliflower with garlic and vinegar sauce

COLIFLOR EN SALSA ROMESCO   boiled cauliflower in peppery sauce

COLINABOS   turnips

CORAZÓN DE ALCACHOFA   arichoke heart

CORAZONES DE MOELLE APIOS   celery hearts braised in stock, with onion puree

CROQUETAS   meat, fish or vegetable croquettes

EJOTES   string beans

ENCURTIDO   pickle

ENDIBIAS   endive

ENDIBIAS BELGAS   Belgian endive, vegetable with long, crispy leaves

ENDIBIAS BRASEADAS   endive braised in butter and water

ENDIBIAS GRATINADAS   endive baked with butter, lemon juice, with grated cheese on top

ENDIBIAS MENIER   endive sauteed with browned butter
and lemon juice
ESCABECHE   pickled
ESCALDÓN   mixed vegetables
ESCALIBADA   eggplant
ESPAÑOLA   with tomatoes
ESPÁRRAGOS   asparagus
ESPÁRRAGOS AMARGUEROS   asparagus with garlic
and paprika
ESPÁRRAGOS ARANGUES FRÍOS   asparagus boiled,
served cold
ESPÁRRAGOS DIFERENTES SALSAS   asparagus with
different sauces
ESPÁRRAGOS DOS SALSAS, CON   asparagus with two
sauces
ESPÁRRAGOS FRÍOS CON SALSA TÁRTARA   cold
asparagus with tartar sauce
ESPÁRRAGOS MANCHEGOS   asparagus with egg yolk
and cumin sauce
ESPÁRRAGOS MAYONESA, CON   cold asparagus with
mayonnaise
ESPÁRRAGOS MIMOSOS   asparagus garnished with
hard egg yolks
ESPÁRRAGOS PARMESANOS   asparagus with melted
butter and grated cheese
ESPÁRRAGOS POLONESES   asparagus boiled, with
chopped eggs, brown butter and bread crumbs
ESPÁRRAGOS SALSA VERDE, CON   asparagus with
green oil and vinegar sauce
ESPÁRRAGOS TRIGUEROS   asparagus pan fried in olive
oil and garlic
ESPIGAS MAÍZ   corn on the cob
ESPINACA   spinach
ESPINACA ANDALUZA   spinach with raisins and pine
nuts
ESPINACA CATALANA   spinach with ham, pine nuts
and garlic

ESPINACA CONCHAS, EN   creamed spinach in a shell

ESPINACA MALAGUEÑA   spinach with raisins and pine nuts

ESPINACA PASAS Y PIÑONES, CON   spinach with raisins and pine nuts

ESPINACA PIÑONES Y ALMENDRAS, CON   spinach with pine nuts and almonds

ESTOFADO QUARESMA, DE   vegetable stew

FAVOS   lima beans

FLAN ALBERGINIES, DE   eggplant flan

FONDAS ALCACHOFAS   artichoke bottoms

FONDOS DE ALCACHOFAS   artichoke bottoms

FONDOS DE ALCACHOFAS PATATAS   sauteed potatoes and artichoke bottoms

FREGINAT   white beans with fried pork liver

FRIJOLADA   bean stew with meats and vegetables

FRIJOLES   beans

FRIJOLES NEGROS   black beans

FRIJOLES REFRITOS   cooked beans, mashed and refried

FRITURA MIXTA   deep-fried meats, chicken, vegetables or fish

GARBANZOS   chick-peas

GARBANZOS CATALANA   chick-peas with tomato sauce

GARBANZOS REFRITOS   refried chick-peas

GRATIN   cooked vegetables or pasta, baked in a casserole with butter, bread crumbs and grated cheese

GRELOS   turnip greens

GUACAMOLE   pureed avocado, onion and seasonings

GUARNICIÓN DE VERDURAS   garnish of vegetables

GUINDILLA   chili pepper

GUISANTES   green peas

GUISANTES AZÚCAR   green peas glazed with butter and sugar

GUISANTES CATALANA   green peas with raisins and pine nuts

GUISANTES CON TOCINO   green peas with sauteed bacon

GUISANTES ESPAÑOLES   green peas sauteed with
   onion, carrot, ham
GUISANTES FRANCESES   green peas with small onions,
   butter and lettuce
GUISANTES GRANADINAS, CON   cooked peas, arti-
   choke hearts, sauteed onions, garlic, tomatoes and
   garnish of poached egg
GUISANTES MANTEQUILLA, CON   buttered peas
GUISANTES MENTA, CON   buttered peas with mint
GUISANTES PAISANOS   green peas with small onions,
   butter and lettuce
GUISANTES REHOGADOS   peas sauteed in butter or oil
GUISANTES SALCHICHAS, CON   green peas with
   sausage, onion, tomato, garlic, mint
GUISANTES SALTEADOS CON JAMÓN   peas sauteed
   with ham
HABAS   broad beans
HABAS ANDALUZA   lima beans with artichoke, cumin
   and eggs
HABAS CATALANA   broad beans with herbs, spices,
   mint, cinnamon
HABAS CON JAMÓN   lima beans or broad beans sauteed
   with wine and ham
HABICHUELAS   kidney beans
HABICHUELAS VERDES   string beans
HINOJO   fennel, a licorice tasting vegetable like celery
HONGO   mushroom
HORTALIZA   greens
HUMITA   corn, tomatoes, green peppers, onion, cheese
JARDINERA   with carrots, peas and mixed vegetables
JUDÍAS   beans
JUDÍAS BLANCAS   white beans
JUDÍAS ESPAÑOLAS   string beans cooked in sauce of
   tomato, onion, garlic flavored olive oil
JUDÍAS PINTAS   pinto beans
JUDÍAS ROJAS   red *or* kidney beans
JUDÍAS VERDES   string beans

JUDÍAS VERDES CON AJO   green beans with butter and
  garlic
JUDÍAS VERDES CON BARCENA   green beans sauteed
  with olive oil and ham
JUDÍAS VERDES CON SALSA DE TOMATE   green beans
  in tomato sauce
JULIANNA   shredded vegetables
LECHUGA   lettuce
LECHUGA BRASEADA CON JUGO   braised lettuce
LEGUMBRE   vegetable
LEGUMBRES RELLENAS   stuffed vegetables
LENTEJAS   lentils
LLENTIE   lentil
LOMBARDA   red cabbage
MAÍZ   corn
MENESTRA ACELGAS, CON   Swiss chard and potato
  casserole with egg crust
MENESTRA LEGUMBRES, CON   mixed vegetable
  casserole
MENESTRA RIOJANA, CON   baked vegetable casserole
MENESTRA VERDURAS, CON   mixed sauteed vegetables
MICHIRONES   lima beans *or* broad beans; also see HABAS
MICHIRONES PICANTICOS   spicy lima beans with
  sausage and chili pepper
MONDONGO   thick vegetable soup or stew
MONJET   black-eyed pea
MONJETAS   dried white beans
MORILLA   morel mushroom
NABOS   turnips
NAVIZA   young turnip greens
NICALOS   wild mushroom
NOPALES   edible cactus
NOPALITO   cactus leaf with salad dressing
OLLA GITANA   vegetable stew
PALMITO   palm heart
PANACHE LEGUMBRES, DE   variety of fresh vegetables
  sauteed together

PANACHE VERDURAS, DE   mixed sauteed vegetables
PATATAS   potatoes
PATATES JUDÍAS VERDES, CON   potato and green bean
    casserole
PELOTAS COCIDAS   stew of meat wrapped in cabbage
    leaves, chicken, pork bacon, chick-peas, potatoes
PENACHO DE LEGUMBRES   mixed sauteed vegetables
PEPINILLOS   gherkins, pickles
PEPINO   cucumber
PIMIENTO   sweet pepper
PIMIENTOS   bell peppers
PIMIENTOS FRITOS   small green peppers fried in olive
    oil with salt
PIMIENTOS MORRÓN   red sweet peppers
PIMIENTOS MORRONES SALTEADOS   sauteed red bell
    peppers
PIMIENTOS RELLENOS   peppers stuffed with rice
PIMIENTOS ROJOS   red bell peppers
PIMIENTOS VERDES   green peppers
PISTO   sauteed eggplant, green peppers and tomatoes,
    served cold
PISTO ARAGONÉS   salt codfish added to the vegetable
    mixture
PISTO BILBAÍNA, DE   ham, squash, peppers, tomatoes,
    onions and garlic cooked together
PISTO ESCABECHE, EN   pickled fish or meat added to
    the vegetable mixture
PISTO MANCHEGO   stew with red and green peppers,
    tomatoes, squash, onion, ham, egg or tuna added
PISTO RIOJANA, CON   stew with tomatoes, eggplant,
    red pepper, onion, garlic, olive oil
POCHAS   dried white beans
POCHAS RIOJANA, CON   white beans cooked with
    garlic, onions, ham and sausage
POROTOS CON GRANADOS   beans with pumpkin and
    corn
POROTOS NEGROS   black beans

PUERRO   leek
PUNTA DE ESPÁRRAGO   asparagus tip
RÁBANO   radish
RÁBANO PICANTE   horse radish
REBOZADAS   vegetables in batter, deep-fried
REMOLACHA   beetroot
REPOLLO   cabbage
ROVELLÓN   wild mushrooms
RUIBARBO   rhubarb
SAMFAINA   half-cooked mixture of eggplant, green
  pepper and tomato
SEPIONES   wild mushrooms
SETAS   mushrooms
SETAS BORDELESA   sauteed in olive oil, garlic, lemon
  juice
SUCULENTO   corn, squash and other vegetables
TOMATES   tomatoes
TOMATES PROVENZAL   tomatoes with garlic flavored
  crumb stuffing, baked
TRUFAS   truffles, a fungus grown underneath the ground
TRUITA SAMFAINA   mixed vegetable omelette
TUMBET   cake of potato and fried eggplant, covered with
  tomato sauce and peppers, then boiled
VERDURAS   vegetables
ZANAHORIAS   carrots
ZANAHORIAS GLASEADAS   carrots glazed with butter
  and sugar
ZANAHORIAS VICHY   carrots glazed with butter and
  sugar with Vichy water
ZARZUELA DE VERDURAS   vegetable stew

Wines, Beers, and Liquors

ABOCADO   sherry from sweet and dry wines
AGUARDIENTE   spirits
AMONTILLADO   medium-dry sherry
ANDALUCÍA   dry sherry and orange juice

ANGÉLICA   herb liqueur
ANÍS   aniseed liqueur
ANÍS DEL MONO   aniseed liqueur
ANÍS SECO   aniseed brandy
ANISADO   slightly alcoholic aniseed based soft drink
APERITIVO   aperitif
BEBIDA   drink
BEBIDA ALCOHÓLICA   alcoholic drink
BOBADILLA DE GRAN RESERVA   wine distilled brandy
BODEGA   wine cellar
BOTELLA   bottle
BURGUNDÍA   burgundy
CALISAYA   quinine flavored liqueur
CARLOS I   wine distilled brandy
CAZALLA   aniseed liqueur
CERVEZA   beer
CERVEZA BARRIL   draft beer
CERVEZA DORADA   light beer
CERVEZA NEGRA   dark beer
CHAMPÁN   sparkling wine
CHICA DE MANZANA   apple brandy
CHINCHÓN   aniseed liqueur
CLARETE   claret
COCKTAIL   cocktail
COINTREAU   orange flavored liqueur
COLA DE MONO   coffee, milk, rum and grape brandy
COÑAC   brandy
CORDONIU   sparkling wine
CORRIENTE   local red wine
COSECHA   vintage of wine
CREMA DE CACAO   cocoa liqueur
CREMAT   liqueur laced cinnamon coffee with heavy cream
CUARENTA Y TRES   egg liqueur
CUBA LIBRE   rum and cola *or* gin and cola
CUERPO   full-bodied
DULCE   sweet
ESPUMOSO   sparkling

FINO   dry sherry
FUNDADOR   wine distilled brandy
GARRAFA   carafe
GINEBRA   gin
GRAND MARNIER   orange flavored liqueur
HIELO   ice
JEREZ   sherry
KIRSCH   white cherry liquor
LICOR   liqueur
LIMONADA MADRILEÑA   red wine, lemon juice, peach
    and lemon wedges and water
LIVIANO   light
MÁLAGA   dessert wine
MANZANILLA   dry white wine
MARGARITA   tequila with lime juice
MEDIA BOTELLA   half bottle
MONTILLA   dessert wine
MOSCATEL   muscatel
MUY SECO   very dry
OLOROSO   sweet, dark sherry
OPORTO   port
PISCO   grape brandy
PONCHE CON COÑAC   hot milk, almond and brandy
    drink
PONCHE CON CREMA   egg-nog liqueur
PULQUE   fermented drink from Mexican plant
RESERVADO   found on Chilean wine labels to indicate
    wine of exceptional quality
RON   rum
SANGRÍA   drink of red wine, orange liqueur and fresh
    fruit pieces
SANGRÍA BLANCA   drink of white wine, orange liqueur
    and fresh fruit pieces
SANGRITA   tequila with tomato, orange and lime juice
SIDRA   cider
SOL Y SOMBRA   blend of brandy and aniseed liqueur
SOLO   straight

SYRUP GRANADINA   pomegranate syrup mixed in wine
  or brandy
TEQUILA   brandy made from aloe plant
TINTO   red wine
TÍO PEPE   a brand name for sherry
TRIPLE SECO   orange liqueur
VASO   glass
VERMU   vermouth
VERMUT   vermouth
VETERANO OSBORNE   wine distilled brandy
VINO   wine
VINO BLANCO   white wine
VINO BURDEOS   bordeaux
VINO CLARETE   rosé wine
VINO COMÚN   table wine
VINO CORRIENTE   local wine
VINO DE LA REGIÓN   local wine
VINO DE MESA   table wine
VINO DEL PAÍS   local wine
VINO DULCE   dessert wine
VINO ESPUMOSO   sparkling wine
VINO ROSADO   rosé wine
VINO SECO   dry wine
VINO SUAVE   sweet wine
VINO TINTO   red wine
XAMPÁÑ   sparkling wine

4

What It Means: A Complete Alphabetical Dictionary of Spanish Food and Drink

A

ABADEJO   codfish
ABOCADO   sherry from sweet and dry wines
ACEDERA   sorrel
ACEDÍAS   flounder
ACEDÍAS FRITAS   pan fried in oil
ACEITE   oil
ACEITUNAS   olives
ACEITUNAS NEGRAS   black olives
ACEITUNAS VERDES   green olives
ACELGAS   Swiss chard
ACELGAS SALTEADAS MIGAS   Swiss chard sauteed
   with croutons
ACHICORIA   chicory
ADEREZO   dressing
ADOBADO   marinated
ADOBO   marinated
AGUA   water
AGUA GASEOSA   soda water
AGUA MINERAL   mineral water
AGUA NATURAL   plain water
AGUACATE   avocado

AGUACATE RELLENO DE GAMBAS CON ADEREZO
avocado filled with prawns in a mayonnaise sauce
AGUARDIENTE   spirits
AGUJA   filled baked pastry
AHUMADO   smoked
AJIACEITE   garlic mayonnaise
AJIACO   meat and potato stew
AJIACO BOGOTANO   chicken soup with potatoes
AJILLO   young garlic
AJO   garlic
AJO ARRIERO   pieces of seafood or fish in a garlic sauce
of tomatoes, bell peppers, hot pepper and olive oil
AJO BLANCO   gazpacho made with oil, almonds and
garlic, cold water, a few grapes
AJO BLANCO CON UVAS   cold soup of almonds, garlic,
vinegar soaked bread, white grapes
AJOLIO   garlic flavored mayonnaise dressing served with
fish
AJOQUESO   melted cheese, peppers, etc.
AL, A LA, A LO   in the style of; as; with
ALASKA LLAMAS   flamed Baked Alaska
ALBAHACA   basil
ALBARICOQUE   apricot
ALBÓNDIGAS   pork meatballs
ALBÓNDIGAS MAYONESA   pork meatballs with mayon-
naise garlic dip
ALBÓNDIGAS SANT CLIMENT   lamb meatballs in rich
brandy sauce
ALBONDIGÓN   meat loaf
ALCACHOFAS   artichokes
ALCACHOFAS ANDALUZAS   artichokes fried with
chopped ham
ALCACHOFAS BORDALESAS   artichokes stewed in
butter with sliced potatoes
ALCACHOFAS POLONESAS   artichokes filled with
chopped egg and crumbs browned in butter

ALCACHOFAS SALTEADAS CON JAMÓN   quartered
  artichokes with diced ham
ALCACHOFAS SERRANO   artichoke quarters with
  Serrano ham
ALCAPARRA   caper
ALFAJORES   filled cookie dessert
ALI-PEBRE   garlic, olive oil and paprika sauce
ALI-OLI   garlic mayonnaise
ALIÑADAS NEGRAS   black olives
ALIÑADAS VERDES   green olives
ALIÑADO   seasoned
ALIÑO   salad dressing with herbs and cheese
ALIOLI   garlic flavored mayonnaise
ALL   garlic
ALLI-PEBRE D'ANGUILES   eel in garlic sauce
ALMEJAS   clams
ALMEJAS AL HORNO   baked stuffed clams
ALMEJAS ARROZ   clams with rice
ALMEJAS ENDIABLADAS   clams in a spicy tomato sauce
ALMEJAS MARINERAS   clams in hot pimento sauce
ALMEJAS ROMESCO   clams in tomato sauce with hot
  pepper, chili pepper, vinegar and garlic
ALMENDRA   almond
ALMENDRA GARRAPINADA   sugared almond
ALMENDRADOS   almond cookies
ALMENDRAS GARRAPIÑADAS   honey glazed almonds
ALMENDRITAS   small squid
ALMÍBAR   syrup
ALMUERZO   lunch *or* mid-morning snack
ALMVERZO   lunch at ten in the morning
ALUBIA   bean
ALUBIAS   small lima beans
ALUBIAS BLANCAS   white lima beans
ALUBIAS ROJAS   red lima beans
ALUBIAS VERDES   green lima beans
ALVERJINES   eggplant

ALVERJINES DULCES   fried eggplant with honey
ALVERJINES FARCIDES ANXOVE   stuffed eggplant with anchovy
AMAICATACO   lunch at eleven in the morning
AMANIDA   salad
AMANIDA BACALLA   salt cod salad
AMANIDA FAVES   bean salad
AMANIDA LLENTIES   lentil salad
AMANIDA MONGETS   black-eyed pea and salt cod salad
AMBAS SALSAS   two sauces of chef's choice
AMEIJOAS CATALANA   steamed clams, sausages, ham and tomatoes
AMETLLE   almond
AMONTILLADO   medium-dry sherry
ANACARDIOS   cashew nuts
ANCAS DE RANA   frog's legs
ANCAS DE RANA A LA PROVENZAL   frog's legs sauteed in olive oil, garlic and parsley
ANCAS DE RANA A LA VALENCIANA   marinated and fried frog's legs
ANCHOA   anchovy
ANCHOVA   anchovy
ANCHOVAS FRITAS   deep-fried anchovies
ANDALUCÍA   dry sherry and orange juice
ANDRAJOS   giblets
ANGÉLICA   herb liqueur
ANGUILA   eel
ANGUILA AHUMADA   smoked eel
ANGULAS   baby eels
ANGULAS BILBAÍNA   sauteed in olive oil with red pepper and garlic
ANGULAS PIL PIL   sauteed in olive oil with red pepper and garlic
ANGULAS VASCA   sauteed in olive oil with red pepper and garlic
ANÍS   aniseed liqueur

ANÍS DEL MONO aniseed liqueur

ANÍS SECO aniseed brandy

ANISADO slightly alcoholic aniseed based soft drink

APERITIVO aperitif

APIOS celery

APIOS BRASEADOS CON TOCINO braised celery with bacon

APIOS MILANESA celery heart casserole with butter and grated cheese, oven-browned

ARENQUE herring

ARENQUE AHUMADO kippered herring

ARENQUE ESCABECHE pickled herring

AREPA corn flapjack

ARLEQUÍN DE FRESA Y VAINILLA ice cream of strawberry and vanilla

ARROCES rice

ARROZ rice

ARROZ ALICANTINO saffron flavored rice with peppers, tomatoes, artichoke hearts and boiled fish

ARROZ AZAFRÁN saffron rice

ARROZ BACALAO, CON rice, codfish, onion, tomato, potato, fish broth, garlic

ARROZ BANDA rice with fish, shellfish, garlic, tomatoes, wine

ARROZ BLANCO boiled rice

ARROZ CALABACÍN rice with zucchini, red pepper, tomato, garlic, green beans

ARROZ CALDERO MURCIANA rice with fish, dried red peppers, garlic, shrimp, squid, tomato, fish broth

ARROZ CATALANA rice, rabbit, sausage, pork ribs, ham and pea pods

ARROZ CORDERO, CON rice with lamb, chick-peas, tomato, bacon, sausage

ARROZ COSTA BRAVA rice with chicken, lobster, bacon, tomatoes, garlic

ARROZ COSTEÑO rice with oven-browned crust, chick-peas, sausages, chicken, garlic, eggs

ARROZ COSTRA   rice with chicken, rabbit, sausages, black pudding, chick-peas topped with meatballs made of pork, hidden under beaten egg, baked in oven to form a crust

ARROZ COSTRA ALICANTINO   rice with meatballs, chicken, sausage, chick-peas, sausage, pork cubes and eggs baked on top

ARROZ COSTRADO HUEVOS   crusted rice with chicken, ham, sausages, chick-peas, onion, eggs

ARROZ CUBANA   oven-cooked rice with fried eggs

ARROZ DOCE   rice pudding

ARROZ ESCARLATA   rice with tomatoes and prawns

ARROZ ESPAÑOLA   rice with chicken liver, pork, tomatoes

ARROZ HORNO, AL   rice, chick-peas, onion, tomato, garlic, potato, sausage

ARROZ LANGOSTA, CON   rice with spiny lobster

ARROZ LECHE ASTURIANO, CON   rice pudding with anisette, cinnamon, boiled down milk, brandy

ARROZ LECHE GALLEGO, CON   rice pudding with caramelized coating

ARROZ LECHE, CON   rice pudding

ARROZ MARINERO   rice with shellfish

ARROZ MARISCOS, CON   rice with shellfish

ARROZ MEJILLONES Y ALMEJAS, CON   rice with mussels and clams

ARROZ MEJILLONES, CON   rice with mussels

ARROZ MIRAMAR   rice, mussels, shrimp, olive oil, pork, ham, onion, squid, firm fish, tomato, artichoke hearts

ARROZ NEGRO   rice with squid, onion, fish broth, tomato, chili pepper, wine

ARROZ PARRILLADO   rice, meats, chicken and vegetables

ARROZ, PATO CON   roast duck with sausage and ham flavored rice

ARROZ POLLITOS, CON   rice with chicken, wine, tomato puree, onion, ham, grated cheese

ARROZ POLLO, CON   rice prepared in broth with chicken

ARROZ PRIMAVERA   rice with spring vegetables
ARROZ ROSEXAT   saffron rice pilaf cooked in a broth,
    served browned with sausages and pork and bacon
    meatballs
ARROZ SANTANDERINO   rice with salmon and milk
ARROZ VALENCIANO   rice with vegetables, chicken,
    shellfish
ARVEJAS PARTIDAS   split peas
ASADAS   roasted
ASADILLO   peppers roasted with garlic, tomato and oil
ASADO   roast
AST   on a spit
ASTURIAS   strong, sharp cheese
ATÚN   tuna fish
ATÚN ESCABECHADO   pickled tuna fish
ATÚN GUIPUZCOANA   fresh tuna, pan fried in oil, wine
    and onions
ATÚN SEVILLANO   fresh tuna fried in butter, marinated
    and simmered in wine, vinegar, garlic, oil and olives
ATÚN VASCO   tuna steaks baked in tomato and wine
AVE   bird
AVE SUPREMA   boneless breast of chicken
AVE SUPREMA PERIGOT   chicken breasts stuffed with
    truffle flavored veal paste, poached in butter
AVELLANA   hazelnut
AVES   poultry
AZAFRÁN   saffron
AZUCADA   sprinkled with sugar
AZÚCAR   sugar

B

BABARRÚA CON NARANJA MORA   frozen orange
    custard with blackberry sauce
BACALAO   dried salt cod fish
BACALAO AJO ARRIERO, CON   pieces of codfish
    braised in oil with garlic, tomatoes, red peppers

BACALAO BATURRA   pieces of cod, cream, garlic and scrambled eggs

BACALAO CASERO   codfish in garlic-oil sauce

BACALAO GOMES SA   salt cod with potatoes and onions

BACALAO LLAUNA   codfish pan-fried with olive oil, garlic, tomatoes, red pepper, wine, then oven-browned

BACALAO NAVARRA   cod braised in garlic sauce, onion, tomato, chili pepper, sliced potatoes, rice and saffron

BACALAO PASAS Y PIÑONES, CON   codfish with raisins and pine nuts

BACALAO PIL PIL   codfish simmered and served in hot garlic olive oil

BACALAO RIOJANO   cod, oven baked in a casserole with sauteed onions and garlic, red bell peppers

BACALAO SALSA VERDE, CON   codfish simmered and served in green sauce of parsley, garlic, vinegar-soaked bread and butter

BACALAO SAMFAINA   cod sauteed in tomato, onion, eggplant, peppers

BACALAO VIZCAÍNA   cod with green peppers, potatoes, tomato sauce

BAJOCA FARCIDES   peppers stuffed with rice, pork, tomatoes and spices

BANDA CON ALMENDRAS   almond and marmalade puff pastry

BANDEJA   tray

BANDERILLAS   toothpicks with bits of delicacies, such as pickled vegetables, ham, cheese, smoked fish

BARBO   river fish

BARCOS DE ANCHOAS   anchovy boat tarts

BARQUILLOS   round cookie pastries

BARTOLILLOS   custard filled fried pastry made with wine, lemon peel, cinnamon

BATATA   sweet potato

BATATAS PORTUGUESAS   Portuguese fried potatoes

BATIDO   milk shake

BEBER   to drink

BEBIDA   a drink
BEBIDA ALCOHÓLICA   alcoholic drink
BECADA   woodcock
BECHAMELLE   creamy white sauce
BEIXAMEL   bechamel sauce
BERBERECHO   small cockle
BERENJENA   eggplant
BERENJENA CON QUESO   eggplant baked with a cheese
    cover
BERENJENA FRITA   eggplant pan fried in oil
BERENJENA PARRILLADA   sliced and grilled eggplant
BERENJENA PROVENZAL   fried eggplant stuffed with
    tomato, garlic, onions, sprinkled with grated cheese and
    baked
BERRAZA   parsnip
BERRO   cress
BERZA   cabbage
BESUGO   sea bream, like red snapper or porgy
BESUGO BILBAÍNO   fish dipped in egg, fried in deep fat
BESUGO DONOSTIARRO   charcoal grilled sea bream fish
BESUGO HORNO, AL   baked red snapper
BESUGO MADRILEÑO   baked porgy in wine tomato
    sauce
BESUGO PIÑONES, CON   porgy sauteed in wine and
    pine nut sauce
BESUGO RELLENO   baked porgy stuffed with egg, ham,
    onion, pimiento
BIEN COCIDO   steak well-done
BIEN HECHO   well-done
BIEN PASADO   well-done
BIFE PORTUGUÉS   garlic rubbed steak, pan fried in olive
    oil
BIFTEC   steak
BISCUIT CON NUECES Y SALSA DE FRAMBUESA   ice
    cream dessert with chopped walnuts and raspberry sauce
BISCUIT GLACE   ice cream dessert
BISCUITS   molded frozen desserts

BISQUE   creamy soup of pureed seafood
BISQUE CON CANGREJOS   bisque with crab
BISQUE CON LANGOSTA   bisque with spiny lobster
BISQUE CON LANGOSTINOS   bisque with large
  prawns
BISQUE HOMARD   bisque with lobster
BISTEC   beefsteak
BISTEC DE TERNERA   veal steak
BIZCOCHA MANCHEGA   cake soaked in milk, sugar,
  vanilla and cinnamon
BIZCOCHITOS   crackers, cookies
BIZCOCHO   cake
BIZCOCHO ALMENDRAS   almond spongecake
BIZCOCHO BORRACHO   spongecake with rum, wine or
  syrup
BIZCOCHO BORRACHO CREMA   liqueur flavored cake
  with custard filling
BIZCOCHO CREMA   spongecake with cream filling
BIZCOCHO GENOVESO   ladyfingers
BIZCOCHOS   sweet biscuits
BIZCOCHOS BORRACHOS   tea cakes with caramelized
  sugar and wine
BIZCOCHUELO   cake
BIZCOTELA   glazed cookie
BLANCO NEGRO   chocolate pudding covered with
  whipped cream
BLANDO   soft
BLEDOS   Swiss chard
BLEDOS PANSES PIÑONES   Swiss chard with raisins
  and pine nuts
BOBADILLA DE GRAN RESERVA   wine distilled brandy
BOCADILLO   sandwich
BOCADILLOS DE MONJA   almond and egg yolk candies
BODEGA   wine cellar
BOGAVANTE   lobster with claws, *or* large crayfish with
  pincers

BOGAVANTE AMERICANA   boiled pieces of lobster or crayfish with sauce of tomatoes, onions, white wine, paprika or mild red pepper, oven browned

BOGAVANTES   large clawed lobster similar to Maine lobster

BOLETA GRAELLA   grilled wild mushroom

BOLINAS DE BACALAO   codfish cakes

BOLLITO   roll

BOLLO   roll *or* cake

BOLO DE ALMENDRA ALGARVIA   almond layer cake

BOLO REY   candied fruit and nut bread

BOMBA   molded frozen dessert

BOMBA MERCEDES   mold with apricot ice and a custard mixture with Chartreuse liquor

BOMBÓN   chocolate

BOMBONES HIGOS   fig candies with almonds

BONITO   striped tuna fish

BONITO MARINERO   tuna fish slices pan-fried in olive oil, with tomato sauce, garlic, onion

BOQUERONES   smelts fish like a large anchovy

BOQUERONES EN VINAGRE   smelts marinated in garlic vinegar

BOQUERONES EN VINAGRE FRITOS   fish marinated in garlic vinegar and fried

BORRACHUELOS   fried pastry with licorice flavor and sesame seeds

BORTSCH POLONESA   Polish red beet soup with other vegetables and sausages

BOTELLA   bottle

BOU   beef

BRANDADA BACALLA   salt cod puree

BRANDADA CARXOFE   salt cod puree with artichoke

BRANDADA DE BACALAO   paste of mashed codfish and boiled potatoes with olive oil and milk

BRASA   cooked over coals

BRASEADO   braised

BRAZO GITANO sponge cake roll with rum cream filling
BRÉCOL broccoli
BREVAS black figs
BREVAS SORIA custard filled small doughnuts
BROA Portuguese cornbread
BROCHETAS skewered
BRÓCULI broccoli
BUDÍN pudding
BUEY ox
BUEYES DE MAR large crabs with pincers
BULLABESA fish soup stew
BULLABESA MARSELLA soup with fish and shellfish,
    garlic, onions, tomatoes
BUÑUELITOS CHORIZO fritters made with chopped
    sausage
BUÑUELITOS DE BACALAO cod fritters
BUÑUELITOS DE HUEVO DURO hard-boiled egg
    fritters
BUÑUELITOS DE JAMÓN ham fritters
BUÑUELITOS DE POLLO chicken fritters
BUÑUELO fritter *or* doughnut
BUÑUELO CON CREMA fried doughnut, filled with
    cream or custard
BUÑUELOS sweet fritters; also see BUNYOL and
    BUÑUELO
BUÑUELOS CON LIMÓN lemon crullers
BUÑUELOS CON MANZANA apple fritters
BUÑUELOS CON PLÁTANO deep-fried banana fritters
BUÑUELOS SAN ISIDRO deep-fried sweet fritters
    custard filled
BUÑUELOS VIENTO deep-fried sweet fritters
BUNYOL fried pastry
BUNYOL DE BACALLA salt cod fritter
BUNYOL DE CIURENY wild mushroom fritter
BURGOS soft, creamy cheese
BURGUNDÍA burgundy
BUTIFARRA spicy sausage

BUTIFARRA Y JUDÍAS   broiled sausage with white beans
BUTIFARRA Y SETAS   baked sausages and mushrooms

C

CABALLA   mackerel-like fish
CABALLA VINAGRETA   lightly broiled, then covered
  with wine vinegar, garlic onion sauce
CABELLO DE ÁNGEL   fine noodles; angel's hair
CABELLOS DE ÁNGEL CALABACÍN   made of pumpkin
  squash, cooked in flavored sugar syrup
CABEZA   head
CABEZA DE TERNERA   calf's head
CABRA   goat
CABRALES   blue cheese
CABRITO   kid
CACA   wild game
CACAHUETE   peanut
CACHELOS   boiled diced potatoes, cabbage, garlic,
  bacon, chorizo sausage
CACHOPO   beef stuffed with ham, asparagus tips,
  breaded and pan fried
CAFÉ   coffee
CAFÉ CORTADO   strong coffee in a small cup with dash
  of milk
CAFÉ DESCAFEINADO   decaffeinated coffee
CAFÉ EXPRES   espresso, small cup of strong black coffee
CAFÉ GRANIZADO   iced coffee with milk
CAFÉ CON LECHE   coffee with milk
CAFÉ NEGRO   black coffee
CAFÉ SIN LECHE   coffee without milk
CAFÉ SOLO   black coffee
CALABACÍN   zucchini *or* squash
CALABACÍN AL HORNO   baked zucchini
CALABACÍN RELLENO   stuffed with meat or other type
  of stuffing
CALABAZA   pumpkin or squash blossoms

CALAMARES   squid
CALAMARES A LA PARRILLA   squid basted with garlic
flavored olive oil and grilled
CALAMARES CON JEREZ   squid casserole with dry
sherry
CALAMARES RELLENOS   squid fried in oil and stuffed
with chopped ham
CALAMARES ROMANOS   squid slices fried in batter
CALAMARES SALTEJATS ALL JULIVERT   squid sauteed
with garlic
CALAMARES TINTOS   squid braised in its own ink
CALCOT FRITAS   deep-fried green onion
CALCOTADA   grilled green onions, spicy sauce
CALDERADA   seafood stew
CALDERETA   stew of kid goat, fried with piquant pep-
pers and seasoned with mashed liver, raw garlic and red
peppers
CALDERETA ASTURIANA   mixed fish stew
CALDERETA DE CABRITO   goat stew in red wine
CALDERETA DE CODORNICES   quail and onions potted
in chicken broth
CALDERETA DE LANGOSTA   lobster, onions, garlic,
tomatoes in fish broth
CALDILLO DE CONGRÍO   conger-eel soup with toma-
toes and potatoes
CALDO   meats or fish, vegetables, soup bones made into
a broth
CALDO COCIDO   liquid part of soup-stew
CALDO COLADO   liquid part of soup-stew
CALDO DE CARNE   beef broth
CALDO DE GALLINA   chicken soup
CALDO DE PERRO GADITANO   fish broth, onion, garlic,
lime juice and orange juice
CALDO DE PESCADO   fish broth
CALDO DE POLLO   chicken soup
CALDO GALLEGO   thick soup stew of cabbage, potatoes,
beans, ham, sausage, spareribs

CALDO GALLEGO BURGUÉS   soup stew of smoked ham and bacon, veal, sausage, chicken, white beans, cabbage, turnips

CALDO GALLEGO CAMPESINO   soup of white beans, smoked ham and bacon, onion, cabbage, turnips

CALDO PARTERO   soup of various meats and vegetables

CALDO VERDE   potato and kale soup with sausage

CALIENTE   hot *or* warm

CALISAYA   quinine flavored liqueur

CALLOS   tripe, stomach lining

CALLOS ANDALUZ   tripe stewed in mint sauce, beans, onion, tomato, pimento, ham and sausage

CALLOS ASTURIANOS   tripe stewed with pig's feet, sausage, ham, bell peppers, onion, hot pepper, garlic, tomato paste and oil

CALLOS GALLEGOS   soup of tripe, chick-peas, sausage, onion, garlic, wine

CALLOS MADRILEÑOS   tripe in a sauce of tomato, onion with black pudding, chorizo and ham

CAMARÓN   shrimp

CAMEMBERT CON JITOMATE CONFITURA   fried camembert with tomato preserves

CAMOTE   sweet potato

CANAILLAS   sea snail

CANAPE   toasted or fried crustless bread covered with a spread

CANAS   fried pastry cylinders filled with cream or custard

CANASTILLA DE FRUTA   small basket of fruit

CANASTILLA FRUTAS   basket of fresh fruit

CANELA   cinnamon

CANELONES   stuffed pasta covered with sauce, grated cheese, baked

CANELONES A LA REINA   pasta with stuffing of chicken and mushrooms with white sauce

CANELONES ROSSINI   pasta with stuffing of ham, bacon, chicken livers, onions and tomatoes, with white sauce

CANGREJO   crab
CANGREJO DE MAR   sea crab with hard shell
CANGREJO DE RÍO   river crayfish
CANGREJOS EN JEREZ   hard shell crabs in dry sherry
CANJA   chicken soup with lemon and mint
CANTARELA   mushroom
CANUTILLOS   baked puff pastry horns filled with
   custard
CAPIROTADA   sweetbread pudding with cinnamon
CAPÓN   castrated roaster chicken
CAPÓN SOUVAROFF   roast stuffed with goose liver,
   braised in pastry
CAQUI   persimmon
CARABINEROS   prawn with red shell
CARACOL   snail
CARAMELO   caramel
CARBONADA   meat stew
CARBONADA CRIOLLA   pumpkin stuffed with beef and
   baked
CARBONADA DE VACA   braised beef in beer with
   tomato puree
CARDO   cardoon, plant resembling artichoke
CARGOLADA   grilled snails
CARLOS I   wine distilled brandy
CARNE   meat
CARNE ASADA AL HORNO   roast meat
CARNE CASTELLANA   slices of beef and ham sauteed in
   onions, garlic, wine and oil
CARNE CERDO, DE   pork
CARNE FUEGO LEÑA   charcoal broiled meats
CARNE MEMBRILLO, DE   sweet fruit paste
CARNE MOLIDA   chopped beef
CARNE PARRILLA, A LA   charcoal grilled steak
CARNE PICADA   chopped beef
CARNE TERNERA   veal
CARNE VACA, DE   beef
CARNE VINO   pork braised in white wine

CARNERO   mutton

CARPA   carp

CARRO   food cart

CASA   of the restaurant

CASADIELLES   baked puff pastry horns filled with walnut mixture

CASATA NAPOLITANA   molded ice cream, with strawberry and praline ice cream, crumbled macaroons, candied fruit, maraschino liqueur

CASERA   home style

CASERO   homemade

CASTAÑA   chestnut

CASTAÑOLA   sea perch

CASTAÑOLA CATALANA   sea perch with onions, tomatoes

CASTELLÓN DE OLLA   stew of white beans, beef and bacon

CATALANA   with onions, parsley and tomatoes

CAZA   game

CAZADORA   with mushrooms, onions, wine

CAZALLA   aniseed liqueur

CAZOLADA   potato and vegetable stew with bacon and ribs

CAZOULET TOLOSANA   casserole with white beans, pork, ham, fresh bacon, sausages and duck meat

CAZUELA   casserole

CAZUELA ARAGONESA   casserole of white beans with sausage

CAZUELA DE CORDERO   casserole of lamb stew with vegetables

CAZUELA DE FIDEOS   noodle dish with beans and cold spices

CAZUELA DE GAMBAS   casserole of prawns simmered in sauce

CAZUELA DE LOMO BUTIFARRA   pork chops and sweet sausage casserole

CAZUELITA   individual casserole

CEBOLLAS   onions
CEBOLLAS RELLENAS   beef stuffed onions with wine,
    cream and cheese
CEBOLLETA   chive
CEBOLLITAS   small onions
CEBOLLITAS RELLENAS   small stuffed onions
CEBÓN   castrated beef
CEBRERO   blue-veined, creamy, sharp cheese
CENA   light supper
CENTOLLO   giant crab, like stone crab
CENTOLLO A LA DONOSTIARRA   crab meat simmered
    in sauce of tomato and cognac served hot in shell
CENTOLLO GALLEGO   crab boiled, served whole,
    cracked, cold
CERDO   pork
CERDO CARRE   bone-in pork loin roast
CERDO, CHULETAS DE   pork chops
CERDO, CINTA DE   loin of pork
CERDO CORTIJERA, A LA   pork braised in olive oil
CERDO ESTERHAZY, FILETE DE   pork browned, pap-
    rika seasoned, simmered in sour cream
CERDO, FILETE DE   pork tenderloin
CERDO, LOMO DE   pork loin
CERDO, LONJA DE   pork loin or pork chop, pan fried
CERDO, MANITAS DE   pigs' feet breaded and pan fried
CERDO NORMANDA, A LA   pork chops in sauce from
    pan juices with cream
CERDO, OLLA DE   pork loin fried in earthenware pot
CERDO ORÉGANO, CON   pork cooked with oregano
CERDO PORTUGUÉS   slices of pork coated with garlic
    paste and browned in white wine and broth
CERDO PROVENZALE, A LA   pork loin seasoned with
    sage and roasted with garlic and olive oil
CERDO RIOJANA, A LA   pork with tomatoes and bell
    peppers
CERDO SARTÉN, EN   roasted pork loin sauteed in butter
CERDO, SOLOMILLO DE   pork tenderloin

CEREZA   cherry
CERVEZA   beer
CERVEZA BARRIL   draft beer
CERVEZA DORADA   light beer
CERVEZA NEGRA   dark beer
CESTA DE FRUTA   basket of fresh fruit
CESTA FRUTAS   basket of fresh fruit
CEVICHE   fish marinated in lemon and lime juice
CHABACANO   apricot
CHALOTE   shallot
CHALUPAS   spicy Mexican dish of sausage, chili, onions
CHAMPÁN   sparkling wine
CHAMPIÑONES   mushrooms
CHAMPIÑONES AJILLO   mushrooms stir-fried in olive
   oil with garlic chili pepper
CHAMPIÑONES BORDALESA, A LA   mushrooms
   sauteed in oil with onion, garlic, lemon juice
CHAMPIÑONES JEREZ, EN   mushrooms sauteed in
   sherry wine
CHAMPIÑONES RELLENOS   pork stuffed baked
   mushrooms
CHAMPIÑONES REVOLTILLOS   scrambled eggs and
   sauteed mushrooms
CHAMPIÑONES SALTEADOS   mushrooms sauteed in
   garlic butter
CHAMPIÑONES SEGOVIANA   mushrooms sauteed in
   wine, garlic and bacon
CHANCHO ADOBADO   pork, sweet potatoes, orange
   and lemon juice
CHANFAINA   goat liver and kidney stew in thick sauce
CHANFAINA SALMANTINA   dish of rice, giblet, lamb
   sweetbread and pieces of chorizo
CHANGURRO   crab meat with sherry and brandy
CHANGURRO VASCO   crab meat simmered in sauce of
   tomato, cognac and served hot in shell
CHANQUETES   small whitebait fish or sardines, deep
   fried

CHATEAUBRIAND   steak from center of filet
CHATEAUBRIAND BUEY MASCOTA   steak sauteed
    with wine and sauce made from pan juices
CHAYOTE   Mexican squash
CHICA DE MANZANA   apple brandy
CHICHARRO   horse mackerel
CHILE   chili pepper
CHILE NOGADO   green peppers stuffed with whipped
    cream and nut sauce
CHILE Y QUESO   spicy chilis and cheese
CHILINDRÓN   thick tomato sauce with ham, red bell
    peppers, oil and garlic
CHILINDRONES   sauce made with pepper, tomato and
    fried onion
CHIMICHURRI   hot parsley sauce
CHINCHÓN   aniseed liqueur
CHIPERONES   squid
CHIPERONES TINTA   squid braised in their own ink
CHIRIVÍA   parsnip
CHIRLAS   small clam
CHOCOLATE   hot milk and chocolate, boiled and
    whipped
CHOCOLATE CON LECHE   hot chocolate with milk
CHOPA   sea bream-like fish
CHORIZO   sausage of pork, pork fat, spices, herbs and
    paprika
CHORIZO CON SIDRA   sausage and apples in hard cider
    sauce
CHORIZO DE OLLA   fried sausage preserved in pork fat
CHORIZO HOJALDRADO   sausage slices baked in pastry
CHORÓN   tomato flavored Bearnaise sauce
CHOTO   bull meat
CHUCRUT   sauerkraut
CHULETAS   cutlet
CHULETAS AÑONO   mutton chops
CHULETAS CARNERO   lamb or mutton chop
CHULETAS CASTELLANA   veal chops browned in lard

CHULETAS CORDERO PARISIENNE, DE   lamb chops grilled with browned potatoes, artichoke bottoms, Madeira sauce

CHULETAS DE CERDO   pork chops

CHULETAS DE CERDO ASTURIANAS   pork chops with apples in cider sauce

CHULETAS DE CERDO CON CIRUELA PASA   pork chops, prunes, cinnamon, wine

CHULETAS DE CERDO CON JEREZ   pork chops with sherry and almonds

CHULETAS DE CERDO CON PIMIENTOS JAMÓN   pork chops sauteed with pimientos, ham, tomato, onions

CHULETAS DE CERDO RIOJANA   pork chops sauteed with pimientos, tomato, onions

CHULETAS DE CORDERO   lamb chops

CHULETAS DE CORDERO A LA NAVARRA   lamb chops and sausages in tomato sauce

CHULETAS DE CORDERO CON ALLIOLI   grilled rib lamb chops with garlic mayonnaise

CHULETAS DE CORDERO ROMESCO   grilled rib lamb chops with peppery sauce

CHULETAS DE CORDERO VILLEROI   lamb fried with brown meat sauce, breaded and fried again

CHULETAS DE PUERCO   pork chops

CHULETAS DE TERNASCO   baby lamb chops

CHULETAS DE TERNERA   veal cutlets

CHULETAS DE TERNERA AJO CABINIL   veal chops sauteed with garlic, vinegar and paprika

CHULETAS DE TERNERA CAZUELA   veal chops braised in sauce with oil, tomatoes and onion

CHULETAS DE TERNERA CON HABAS   veal chops with lima beans in onion, tomato sauce

CHULETAS DE TERNERA HORTELANAS   veal chops with ham, mushrooms and finely chopped vegetables

CHULETAS HOLSTEIN   veal cutlets topped with egg

CHULETAS PAPILLOTE   veal chops sauteed in butter with chopped mushrooms, sealed in paper and oven baked

CHULETAS VILLAGODIO   rib steak with bone in
CHULETAS ZINGARA, A LA   cutlets sauteed in butter
  with Marsala wine and mushroom sauce
CHULETÓN   large rib steak
CHUMBO   prickly pear
CHUPE   thick soup or stew, usually with fish
CHUPE DE MARISCOS   scallops with creamy sauce and
  cheese
CHURRASCO   charcoal grilled meat, generally beef
CHURRO   deep-fried doughnut
CHURRO MADRILEÑO   crisp fried cruller
CIERVO   deer, venison
CIGALAS   sea crayfish with claws, like Maine lobster
CIGALAS COCIDAS   boiled crayfish
CINCHO   hard cheese
CIRUELA   plum
CIRUELA PASA   prune
CIURENY   wild mushrooms
CIVET   deer stew with onions and mushrooms
CIVET LLAGOSTA   lobster stew
CLARETE   claret
CLAUDIA   greengage plum
COCA   open face baked pie with vegetable or meat
  topping
COCA DE ANEE OLIVES   duck and olive pastry
COCAO   cocoa
COCHIFRITO   fricassee of lamb
COCHIFRITO DE CORDERO   lamb or kid stew
COCHIFRITO NAVARRO   small pieces of fried lamb
COCHINILLO   roast pig
COCHINILLO ASADO   roast suckling pig
COCHINILLO SEGOVIANO   suckling pig in clay oven,
  baked with wine
COCIDA   boiled
COCIDO   a boiled dinner of soup, vegetables, meat,
  bacon, black pudding, chick-peas
COCIDO AL VAPOR   steamed

COCIDO ANDALUZ   beef, pork, sausage, squash, green beans, garlic cooked into a soup-stew

COCIDO MADRILEÑO   a soup-stew of chick-peas, veal or beef, ham, salt pork, potatoes, sausage, cabbage, chicken, carrots, onions, pig's foot and garlic

COCIDO PORTUGUÉS   boiled meats, chicken and vegetables

COCINA   kitchen; cuisine

COCKTAIL   cocktail

COCO   coconut

CÓCTEL DE CAMARONES   shrimp cocktail

CÓCTEL DE FRUTA   fruit cocktail

CÓCTEL DE GAMBAS   prawn cocktail

CÓCTEL DE MARISCOS   cocktail of various seafoods

CODORNICES   quail

CODORNICES ASADAS EN HOJAS DE UVA   quail baked, wrapped in grape leaves

CODORNICES CEREZAS, CON   quail braised with cherries

CODORNICES ESCABECHE, EN   grilled or roasted quail in a marinade

CODORNICES ESTOFADAS   braised quail with onion, garlic, wine and brandy

CODORNICES HIDO   quail done in brandy and wine, onion, pepper, served in a nest of French fried potatoes

CODORNICES, PAREJA DE   two braised quail in sauce

CODORNICES PERIGOURDINE   quail casserole roasted with Madeira flavored gravy

CODORNICES POCHAS CALZADAS   quail with lima beans, onion, tomato, sausage

CODORNICES UVAS, CON   quail poached with peeled grapes, wine flavored aspic

CODORNICES ZURRÓN   quail wrapped in ham, inside green pepper with tomatoes and onions

CODORNIZ   quail

COINTREAU   orange flavored liqueur

COL   cabbage

COL DE BRUSELAS   Brussels sprouts

COL DE BRUSELAS SALTEADO   sauteed Brussels sprouts

COL FERMENTADA   sauerkraut

COLA   tail

COLA ANDALUZA   braised tail with potatoes, onion, garlic, tomato

COLA DE MONO   coffee, milk, rum and grape brandy

COLA DE TORO   bull's tail braised in gravy with onion, cabbage, carrots, bacon and sausage

COLAS DE CIGALA   crayfish tails

COLIFLOR   cauliflower

COLIFLOR CON AJO ARRIERO   deep-fried cauliflower with garlic and vinegar sauce

COLIFLOR EN SALSA ROMESCO   boiled cauliflower in peppery sauce

COLINABOS   turnips

COMER   to eat

COMIDA   main meal of the day

COMPOTA   stewed fruit

COMPOTAS   fruits preserved in syrup

CON   with

COÑAC   brandy

CONCHA   shell used as serving dish

CONCHAS FINAS   medium size clams

CONDIMENTO   relish

CONEJO   rabbit

CONEJO ALIOLI, CON   broiled rabbit, baked in wine garlic sauce

CONEJO AMPURDANESO   rabbit braised in broth with onion, tomato and rabbit liver paste, chocolate, garlic, pepper and almonds

CONEJO CASERO   rabbit braised in wine, onion, mushrooms, bacon and lard

CONEJO CAZADOR   rabbit casserole, flamed in brandy with onion, wine, tomato, mushrooms

CONEJO CIRUELAS Y PIÑONES, CON   sauteed rabbit with prunes and pine nuts

CONEJO JUANA, A LA   baked rabbit with tomatoes, garlic, onion, olive oil, almonds, cognac

CONEJO, MUSLO DE   roasted rabbit thigh

CONEJO PEPITORIA, A LA   baked rabbit with egg, lemon sauce and mushrooms

CONEJO ALIOLI, PIERNA DE   broiled rabbit leg with garlic mayonnaise

CONEJO PIRINEO   rabbit casserole with onion, wine, pine nuts, almond and garlic

CONEJO SALMANTINO   rabbit potted with onion, garlic, vinegar, olive oil, pepper

CONEJO SOBRE BRASAS   rabbit broiled over charcoal

CONEJO THEBUSSEM   braised pieces of rabbit with a sauce of oil, bread and ground almonds

CONEJO TOMATE, CON   rabbit marinated in wine, sauteed in wine, onion, garlic, red pepper

CONEJO VINO BLANCO, CON   rabbit sauteed in butter, simmered in a casserole with white wine

CONFITURA   jam

CONGELADO   frozen

CONGRI MUSSOLINA ALL   chick-peas with garlic hollandaise sauce

CONGRÍO   sea eel, served in sauce of tomato, garlic and oil

CONILL   rabbit

CONSERVA   canned

CONSOMÉ   clear broth of meat, chicken or other stock

CONSOMÉ AVE, DE   chicken and vegetable soup

CONSOMÉ COLBERT   consommé garnished with vegetables and poached egg

CONSOMÉ CRECI   consommé with pureed carrots and rice

CONSOMÉ DE POLLO   chicken and vegetable soup

CONSOMÉ DOBLE   double strength consommé

CONSOMÉ EUGENIA MONTIJO   consommé with truffle and slices of chicken breast poured over egg yolk

CONSOMÉ FIDEOS, DE   consommé with thin spaghetti

CONSOMÉ GELATINOSO   jellied consommé

CONSOMÉ GIRONDINE   beef consommé with ham and carrot strips

CONSOMÉ JEREZ, CON   chicken broth with sherry

CONSOMÉ JULIENNE   consommé with thin strips of cooked vegetables

CONSOMÉ MADRILEÑA, A LA   consommé with tomato pulp

CONSOMÉ MANZANA, DE   apple consommé

CONSOMÉ MOSCOVITA   cold consommé with caviar and whipped cream

CONSOMÉ NATURAL   plain consommé

CONSOMÉ PARMESANO   consommé with Parmesan cheese

CONSOMÉ PROFITEROLES, CON   consommé with filled or unfilled pastry shells

CONSOMÉ SIMPLE   plain broth

CONSOMÉ SOLERA   consommé with sherry

CONSOMÉ TAZA, EN   consommé in a cup

CONSOMÉ TRES FILETES, CON   consommé with tongue, chicken and truffles

CONSOMÉ YEMA, CON   consommé with beaten egg yolks and flour, minced chicken

CONTRA FILETE   boneless loin of beef

CONTRA TERNERA   veal loin steak

COPA ALEJANDRA   mixed fruits in kirsch liquor with strawberry ice cream and strawberries

COPA AMERICANA   pineapple ice with crushed pineapple and macaroons, covered with whipped cream and crystallized fruits

COPA MELBA   poached peach and vanilla ice cream, covered with raspberry sauce and whipped cream

COPA NURIA   whipped eggs served with jam

COPA PEÑASANTA   Baked Alaska for one

COPA VENUS   vanilla ice cream with poached peach, strawberry and whipped cream

COPAS   ice cream sundaes

COQUE   pizza

COQUINAS   small clams

CORAZÓN DE ALCACHOFA   artichoke heart

CORAZONADA   heart stew

CORAZONES DE MOELLE APIOS   celery hearts braised in stock, with onion puree

CORBINA   sea bass *or* perch

CORDERO   lamb

CORDERO ASADO   baby lamb roasted over coals

CORDERO ASADO CASTELLANO   oven roasted lamb with garlic, onion, cumin, oregano

CORDERO ASADO MANCHEGO   roast lamb with garlic, cognac, olive oil, black pepper

CORDERO ASADO SEPULVEDANO   roast lamb in garlic vinegar wine sauce

CORDERO, BRAZUELO DE   roasted front leg of lamb

CORDERO, CALDERETA DE   lamb stew

CORDERO CHILINDRÓN   fried lamb chunks with peppers and tomatoes

CORDERO VILLEROI, CHULETAS DE   fried lamb chops with brown meat sauce, breaded and fried again

CORDERO CHULETAS GUÉRNICA   lamb chops breaded and pan fried

CORDERO CHULETAS NAVARRA   lamb chops sauteed then braised in tomato sauce and onion

CORDERO CHULETAS PARISIENNE   lamb chops grilled with browned potatoes, artichoke bottoms, Madeira sauce

CORDERO, CHULETAS DE   lamb chops; also see CHULETAS

CORDERO COCHIFRITO   sautee of lamb with garlic and lemon

CORDERO, COSTILLAS DE   lamb rib chops

CORDERO, ESPALDA DE   roasted boned and stuffed lamb shoulder

CORDERO GUISADO   lamb stew

CORDERO LECHAL   milk-fed lamb

CORDERO, MANITAS DE   stewed lamb's feet

CORDERO MENESTRA   lamb and vegetable soup-stew
CORDERO MENUDILLOS   internal organs, sauteed
CORDERO PASCUAL   mutton
CORDERO, PATA DE   roasted leg of lamb
CORDERO RECENTAL   spring lamb
CORDERO RIOJANA   stewed with pepper, tomato, garlic
   and oil
CORDON BLEU   slices of veal, slice of ham and Swiss
   cheese, breaded and fried
CORDONIU   sparkling wine
COREGONO LAGO DE CONSTANZA   felchen from
   Lake Constance
CORONA CORDERO   crown of lamb
CORRIENTE   local red wine
CORTADILLO   small pancake
CORTE   slice of
CORZO   deer
CORZO AUSTRIAZA   roasted deer with caraway seeds
CORZO SOLOMILLO   filet or loin of deer
COSECHA   vintage of wine
COSQUERA   fish sauteed in olive oil with garlic, braised
   with wine, clams, peas and asparagus
COSTILLA   lamb rib or chop; also see CHULETAS
COSTILLA DE ADÁN   charcoal broiled beef rib steak
COSTILLA DE CORDERO   lamb chop
COSTILLA GALLEGA   broiled veal chop
COSTILLAS DE CERDO   spareribs
COTELETA   cutlet; also see CHULETAS
COTZE   mussel
CREMA   cream
CREMA BATIDA   whipped cream
CREMA CATALANA   cream custard with cinnamon or
   candied sugar coating
CREMA CATALANA CON CARAMELO   baked custard
   with burned caramel crust
CREMA DAMA BLANCA   vanilla ice cream

CREMA DAMA DIABLO TÚNICA   vanilla ice cream with chocolate sauce

CREMA DAMA PURPÚREO   vanilla ice cream with strawberry sauce

CREMA DE CACAO   cocoa liqueur

CREMA ESPAÑOLA   gelatin and egg dessert

CREMA INGLESA   frothy cooked custard

CREMA JEREZ, DE   chocolate sherry chiffon pudding

CREMA NARANJA, DE   orange cream custard

CREMA NIEVE, DE   beaten egg yolk, sugar and rum

CREMA PASTELERA RON   rum cream filling

CREMA QUEMADA   caramelized custard filling

CREMA   creamed soup with pureed vegetables, seafood, meat, chicken or fish

CREMA AVE, DE   cream of chicken soup

CREMA CARDENAL, DE   lobster soup with added cream

CREMA CAROLINA   cream of chicken soup with cream and cooked rice added

CREMA CARRAMARES, DE   crab bisque with shrimp, onion, carrots, leek, tomato

CREMA CHAMPINOÑES, DE   cream of mushroom soup

CREMA CULTIVADORA   vegetable soup with bacon

CREMA DE POLLO   cream of chicken soup

CREMA ESPÁRRAGOS, DE   cream of asparagus soup

CREMA ESPINACAS, DE   cream of spinach soup

CREMA FAVES, DE   cream of bean soup

CREMA GALLINA, DE   cream of chicken soup

CREMA GUISANTES, DE   cream of pea soup

CREMA LADY CURZÓN   turtle soup with curry powder and whipped cream

CREMA LANGOSTA, DE   cream of spiny lobster soup

CREMA LEGUMBRES, DE   cream of vegetable soup

CREMA MARISCOS, DE   cream of seafood soup

CREMA PRINCESA   cream soup with pieces of chicken breast and asparagus

CREMA REINA   cream of chicken soup

CREMA SOLERA   cream soup with sherry
CREMA SOLFERINO   pureed tomato and potato soup
CREMA ST. GERMÁN   cream of pea soup
CREMA TOMATE, DE   cream of tomato soup
CREMA PERDIZ   cream of partridge soup
CREMAT   liqueur laced cinnamon coffee with heavy
    cream
CREPES   thin filled pancake with creamy sauce
CREPES CREMA   custard filled pancakes
CREPES SUZETTE   pancakes spread with filling flavored
    with orange juice, Cointreau, flamed with cognac
CRIADILLAS DE TORO   bull testicles
CROCANTI   chopped almonds in caramel
CROQUETAS   meat, fish or vegetable croquettes
CROQUETAS DE GALLINA   chicken croquettes
CROQUETAS GAMBAS, DE   fried balls of shrimp
    croquettes
CROQUETAS PAELLA, EN   fried balls of paella rice
    mixture
CROQUETAS POLLO, DE   chicken croquettes
CROQUETES LLAGOSTA, DE   lobster croquettes
CRUDO   raw
CRUSTACEOS   shellfish
CUAJADA LECHE   junket of ewe's milk
CUAJADA MIEL   rennet pudding with honey and
    walnuts
CUARENTA Y TRES   egg liqueur
CUBA LIBRE   rum and cola *or* gin and cola
CUBIERTO   cover charge
CUCHARA   spoon
CUCHARITA   teaspoon
CUCHIFRITO   milk-fed suckling pig
CUCHILLO   knife
CUENTA, POR FAVOR   check, please
CUERPO   full-bodied
CURANTO   seafood, vegetables and pig cooked in an
    earthen well

D

DAMASCO   kind of apricot
DÁTIL   date
DE LA ESTACIÓN   in season
DE, DEL, DE LA   of
DENTÓN   flat fish similar to pompano
DENTÓN MALLORQUINA   deep-fried fish with sauce of oil, garlic and sherry
DESAYUNO   breakfast
DESPUÉS   after
DÍA   of the day
DINERO   money
DON SUERO   ham stuffed veal cutlet
DORADA   fish similar to bream
DOS SALSAS   with two sauces on the side
DUELOS QUEBRANTOS   scrambled eggs with bacon and sausage
DULCE   sweet
DULCE DE MEMBRILLO   quince marmalade
DURAZNO   peach

E

EJOTES   string beans
ELECCIÓN   method of cooking to your choosing
EMBUCHADO   pork sausage
EMBUTIDO   spicy sausage
EMPANADA   meat or fish pie baked with onion and peppers
EMPANADA ASTURIANA   baked sausage pie
EMPANADA BERBERECHA   baked clam pie
EMPANADA BONITA   baked tuna pie
EMPANADA DE LOMO   baked pork pie
EMPANADA DE SARDINAS   baked sardine pie
EMPANADA GALLEGA   chicken filled pastry
EMPANADA HORNO, AL   pastry with minced meat filling

EMPANADILLAS   small fried stuffed pastry turnovers
EMPANADILLAS DE ATÚN   small fried tuna stuffed
   pastry turnovers
EMPANADILLAS DE CHORIZO   chorizo sausage
   pastries
EMPANADILLAS JAMÓN   ham pastries
EMPANADILLAS VALENCIANAS   pastries stuffed with
   ham and tuna
EMPAREDADO   sandwich
EMPAREDADO CALIENTE   hot sandwich like French
   toast with ham filling
EMPERADOR   swordfish
EN   in
EN SU JUGO   in its own juice
ENCEBOLLADA   cooked with sauteed onions
ENCEBOLLADO DE PESCADO   grilled fish covered with
   chopped onions, oil and vinegar
ENCHILADA   Mexican stuffed cornmeal pancake
ENCHILADA ROJA   cornmeal pancake filled with sau-
   sage dipped in red sweet pepper sauce
ENCHILADA VERDE   cornmeal pancake stuffed with
   poultry or meat and braised in a green tomato sauce
ENCURTIDO   pickle
ENDIBIAS   endive
ENDIBIAS BELGAS   Belgian endive, vegetable with long,
   crispy leaves
ENDIBIAS BRASEADAS   endive braised in butter and
   water
ENDIBIAS GRATINADAS   endive baked with butter,
   lemon juice, with grated cheese on top
ENDIBIAS MEUNIERE   endive sauteed with browned
   butter and lemon juice
ENELDO   dill
ENSAIMADA   baked, sugar topped, snail shaped sweet
   rolls
ENSALADA   salad; also see ENTREMESES

ENSALADA ALMORAINA   salad with escarole, tomato, cumin, olive oil and wine vinegar

ENSALADA ANGUILAS, DE   salad with baby eels in garlic, olive oil and vinegar

ENSALADA APIO BLANCO, DE   salad with celery

ENSALADA ARENQUE, DE   herring salad

ENSALADA ARROZ, DE   salad with rice, mushrooms, oil, vinegar, garlic, anchovy, mustard

ENSALADA AVE, DE   chicken salad

ENSALADA BERROS, DE   watercress salad

ENSALADA BLANCA   salad with white beans, onion, oil and vinegar

ENSALADA CORAZÓN DE PALMITO, DE   salad with canned heart of palm

ENSALADA CATALANA   salad with lettuce, onions, bell peppers, tomato, tuna, codfish, ham, sausage, hard-boiled egg

ENSALADA CATALINA   summer salad of romaine or curly endive lettuce, tomatoes, sweet raw onion, green and red peppers, green and black olives

ENSALADA CHAMPIÑÓN   mushroom and ham salad

ENSALADA COLAS DE CANGREJO, DE   crayfish salad

ENSALADA COMÚN   green salad

ENSALADA CORRIENTE   salad of seasonal local ingredients

ENSALADA ENDIVIAS QUESO Y CABRALES, CON   endive salad with blue cheese

ENSALADA ESCALIBADA   artichoke, eggplant, pepper and tomato salad

ENSALADA ESCAROLAS, DE   salad with slightly bitter green head lettuce

ENSALADA ESPARTEROS, DE   salad with tuna, egg, potato, onion, capers

ENSALADA FRUTAS, DE   fruit salad

ENSALADA ILUSTRADA   salad with combination of ingredients

ENSALADA ITALIANA   Italian salad

ENSALADA JUDÍAS VERDES A LA VINAGRETA, DE
salad with green bean, onion, oil and vinegar

ENSALADA KOSH KERA   salad with fish, lobster,
pimiento, olives, eggs, oil and vinegar

ENSALADA LANGOSTA, DE   spiny lobster salad

ENSALADA LEGUMBRES, DE   mixed vegetable salad

ENSALADA MADRILEÑA   salad with lettuce, tomatoes,
hard-boiled eggs, olive oil, vinegar

ENSALADA MIXTA   mixed salad

ENSALADA MURCIANA   salad with romaine lettuce,
green peppers, cucumbers, tomatoes, onion, oil, vinegar

ENSALADA NACIONAL   potato salad with peas, tuna,
ham, pimento

ENSALADA NARANJA Y QUESO, CON   salad with
oranges and cheese

ENSALADA NIÇOISSE   salad with cooked and raw
vegetables, marinated in oil and vinegar, topped with
eggs, anchovies, tuna on a bed of lettuce

ENSALADA NORMAL   green salad

ENSALADA PAÍS, DEL   salad of seasonal local
ingredients

ENSALADA PALMERA, DE   salad of canned palm heart

ENSALADA PATATA Y REMOLACHA, DE   potato and
beet salad

ENSALADA PATATAS, DE   boiled potato salad

ENSALADA PEPINO, DE   cucumber salad

ENSALADA PIPARRADA   cucumber tomato and pepper
salad

ENSALADA POLLO, DE   chicken salad

ENSALADA PRIMAVERA   spring salad with vegetables

ENSALADA RAQUEL   boiled potatoes, artichokes,
asparagus, celery, truffles with mayonnaise dressing

ENSALADA REMOLACHA, DE   red beet salad

ENSALADA RUSA   salad with cooked vegetables in
mayonnaise sauce

ENSALADA SAN ISIDRO   mixed salad of onion, lettuce and tuna

ENSALADA SEVILLANA   salad with curly endive, tarragon, pitted olives, oil and vinegar

ENSALADA SURTIDA   mixed salad

ENSALADA TOMATE Y HUEVO, DE   salad with tomato and egg wedges, onion and vinegar

ENSALADA TOMATES, DE   tomato salad

ENSALADA VALENCIANA   green pepper, lettuce and orange salad

ENSALADA VARIADA   mixed green salad

ENSALADA VERDURAS, DE   vegetable salad

ENSALADA WALDORF   apples, celery, walnut, mayonnaise salad

ENSALADA ZARINA   salad with cooked potatoes, carrots, turnips, topped with cold salmon, lettuce, tomatoes and hard-boiled egg, mayonnaise sauce

ENSALADILLA   mixed vegetable salad

ENSALADILLA RUSA   cooked potato and vegetable salad covered with mayonnaise

ENTRADA   entree, main course

ENTRADAS   light appetizers

ENTRANTES   appetizers

ENTRECOTE   boneless beef rib steak

ENTRECOTE ANGLAISE   beef steak grilled with bacon and potatoes

ENTRECOTE BORDALES   beef steak pan fried in sauce of juices, shallots, bone marrow and wine

ENTRECOTE CEBÓN, DE   beef from fattened steer

ENTRECOTE CECILIA   beef grilled with mushroom, creamed green asparagus tips and puffed potato chips

ENTRECOTE FAVORITO   beef pan fried with sauteed goose liver

ENTRECOTE GUARNICIÓN, DE   beef grilled or pan fried

ENTRECOTE HOSTAL   beef pan fried with sauce from boiled down pan juices, wine and meat

ENTRECOTE MARCHAND VINS   beef grilled and
covered with wine and meat concentrate sauce
ENTRECOTE PIMIENTA   steak with crushed pepper-
corns, pan fried in butter, served in sauce of pan juices,
butter, shallots and cognac
ENTRECOTE PIZZAIOLA   beef pan fried with pan juices,
garlic, tomatoes and oregano in oil
ENTRECOTE QUESO Y CABRALES, CON   boneless beef
tenderloin sauteed with blue cheese, wine, garlic
ENTRECOTE TIROLESA   beef broiled with French fried
onion rings
ENTREMESES   hors-d'oeuvres, first courses
ENTREMESES CORRIENTES   appetizers of seasonal local
ingredients
ENTREMESES DE MAR   seafood appetizers
ENTREMESES DEL MESÓN   appetizers of the restaurant
ENTREMESES DEL PUERTO   seafood appetizers
ENTREMESES ESPECIALES   appetizers as specialties of
the restaurant
ENTREMESES SURTIDOS   assorted appetizers
ENTREMESES VARIADOS   assorted cold appetizers
ERIZO MAR   sea urchin
ESCABECHE   pickled
ESCABECHE GALLINA   chicken marinated in vinegar
ESCABECHE SARDINES   pickled sardines
ESCALDÓN   mixed vegetables
ESCALFADOS   poached eggs
ESCALIBADA   eggplant
ESCALOPE   boneless meat, usually veal
ESCALOPE BOLOGNÉS   veal breaded, fried with ham
and Parmesan cheese, oven melted
ESCALOPE EN CACEROLA   veal sauteed in earthenware
dish with sauce from pan juices
ESCALOPE GUÉRNICA   veal breaded and fried in olive
oil
ESCALOPE HOLSTEIN   veal pan fried, topped with a
fried egg

ESCALOPE MARSALA   veal fried in oil, served in sauce from pan juices and Marsala wine

ESCALOPE MILANÉS   veal dipped in egg, bread crumbs, grated Parmesan cheese and fried

ESCALOPE NAPOLITANO   veal sauteed in butter, coated with sauce, grated cheese, breaded and fried

ESCALOPE NARANJA, CON   veal sauteed in oil, butter and orange juice

ESCALOPE VIENÉS   veal breaded and fried with anchovy butter

ESCALOPE ZÍNGARO   veal sauteed in butter, Marsala wine, mushrooms and served in sauce from pan juices

ESCALOPINES MADRILEÑOS   veal medallions in onion tomato sauce

ESCAROLA   endive

ESCOCIA   codfish

ESCOMBRO   mackerel

ESCUDELLA   soup *or* stew

ESCUDELLA DE PAJES   peasant soup stew

ESCUDELLA PAYES   soup-stew of meats, sausage, cabbage, garbanzo beans, potatoes, vegetables

ESPADÓN   swordfish

ESPADÓN AHUMADO   smoked swordfish

ESPAGUETIS   spaghetti

ESPALDA   shoulder

ESPAÑOLA   with tomatoes

ESPÁRRAGOS   asparagus

ESPÁRRAGOS AMARGUEROS   asparagus with garlic and paprika

ESPÁRRAGOS ARANGUES FRÍOS   asparagus boiled, served cold

ESPÁRRAGOS DIFERENTES SALSAS   asparagus with different sauces

ESPÁRRAGOS DOS SALSAS, CON   asparagus with two sauces

ESPÁRRAGOS FRÍOS CON SALSA TÁRTARA   cold asparagus with tartar sauce

ESPÁRRAGOS MANCHEGOS   asparagus with egg yolk
and cumin sauce

ESPÁRRAGOS MAYONESA, CON   cold asparagus with
mayonnaise

ESPÁRRAGOS MIMOSOS   asparagus garnished with
hard egg yolks

ESPÁRRAGOS MONTAÑESES   asparagus with calves'
tails

ESPÁRRAGOS PARMESANOS   asparagus with melted
butter and grated cheese

ESPÁRRAGOS POLONESES   asparagus boiled, with
chopped eggs, brown butter and bread crumbs

ESPÁRRAGOS SALSA VERDE, CON   asparagus with
green oil and vinegar sauce

ESPÁRRAGOS TRIGUEROS   asparagus pan fried in olive
oil and garlic

ESPASA   swordfish

ESPECIALIDADES   specialties

ESPECIALIDADES CASA   specialties of the restaurant

ESPECIALIDADES DE LA REGIÓN   specialties of the
region

ESPECIE   spice

ESPIGAS MAÍZ   corn on the cob

ESPINACA   spinach

ESPINACA ANDALUZA   spinach with raisins and pine
nuts

ESPINACA CATALANA   spinach with ham, pine nuts
and garlic

ESPINACA CONCHAS, EN   creamed spinach in a shell

ESPINACA MALAGUEÑA   spinach with raisins and pine
nuts

ESPINACA PASAS Y PIÑONES, CON   spinach with
raisins and pine nuts

ESPINACA PIÑONES Y ALMENDRAS, CON   spinach
with pine nuts and almonds

ESPUMA CHOCOLATE   frothy chocolate pudding

ESPUMOSO   sparkling

ESQUEIXADA   shredded salt cod salad
ESQUEIXADA LLUC CAVIAR   marinated hake salad
  with caviar
ESQUEIXADA POLLASTRE   shredded chicken salad
ESQUILAS   prawns
ESTILO   style
ESTOFADO   stew
ESTOFADO BOU   beef stew
ESTOFADO CIRUELAS Y PIÑONES, CON   beef stew
  with prunes and pine nuts
ESTOFADO PATATAS, CON   beef stew with potatoes
ESTOFADO QUARESMA, DE   vegetable stew
ESTOFADO TORO, DE   stew of bull meat, onion, garlic,
  tomatoes, wine, cognac
ESTOFADO VACA, DE   beef stew
ESTRAGÓN   tarragon
ESTRELLADOS   fried eggs
ESTURIÓN   sturgeon
ESTURIÓN CATALANO   sturgeon braised in onion,
  garlic, olive oil

F

FABADA   pork, bean, bacon and sausage stew
FABADA ASTURIANA   stew of large white beans, with
  ham or bacon, sausage, salt pork, onions, garlic and
  saffron
FABADA CON ALMEJAS   soup of white beans, onion,
  garlic, chili pepper, carrots, wine, clams
FAISÁN   pheasant
FAISÁN ALCÁNTARO   pheasant stuffed with liver, wild
  mushrooms, marinated in port wine and roasted
FAISÁN CREMA, CON   pheasant roasted with onions,
  served with sauce of roasting juices and cream
FAISÁN SOUVAROFF   pheasant stuffed with sauteed
  goose liver, roasted in earthenware pot with Madeira
  wine

FAISÁN UVAS, CON   pheasant poached in veal stock and serving cold with wine flavored aspic

FAISÁN UVAS, CON   pheasant poached in veal stock and served cold with wine flavored aspic

FARCELLETS   cabbage dumplings *or* rolled meat

FARCELLETS COL   pork and cabbage dumplings

FARINATOS   sausage which is fried and served with eggs

FATIAS CHINAS   egg and almond slices in syrup

FAVOS   lima beans

FAYULES   flat cakes

FETGE   calf's liver

FETGE CEBA   calf's liver with onion

FIAMBRES   cold cuts of meat

FIAMBRES SURTIDOS   assorted meat cold cuts

FIAMBRES VARIADOS   assorted meat cold cuts

FIDEO   thin noodle

FIDEOS   some form of pasta

FIDEOS DE CAZUELA   noodles with spareribs, sausages, ham and bacon

FIDEOS GORDOS   large noodles

FIGOS RECHEADOS   dried figs stuffed with almonds and chocolate

FIGUES   figs

FILETE   steak

FILETE BUEY   steer

FILETE EMPANADO   skillet fried breaded beef steak

FILETE HORTELANO   steak served with fresh vegetables

FILETE LENGUADO EMPANADO, DE   breaded filet of sole

FILETE LOMO, DE   tenderloin steak

FILETE MECHADO   steak wrapped with pork fat and roasted

FILETE PARRILLA, A LA   grilled steak

FILETE RES, DE   beefsteak

FILETE STROGANOFF   beef cooked in sour cream gravy with onions and mushrooms

FILETE TERNERA, DE   veal tenderloin

FILETE VEDELLA SAMFAINA, DE   roast veal filet with mixed vegetables

FILETE VEDELLA, DE   roast veal filet

FILLOAS CON CREMA   thin dessert pancake filled with custard

FINO   dry sherry

FLAMBÉ   flamed with brandy or cognac

FLAMENCA   with green peppers, onions, tomatoes, peas and sausage

FLAMENQUINES   pork and ham slices fried and served in white sauce

FLAN   dessert of egg custard with caramel sauce

FLAN ALBERGINIES, DE   eggplant flan

FLAN CARAMELO, CON   caramelized baked custard

FLAN CASERO   homemade egg custard

FLAN COCO, DE   caramelized coconut custard

FLAN CREMOSO   boiled custard

FLAN DOBLE   double portion of flan

FLAN GRAN FLANERO   caramel custard

FLAN HUEVO, DE   egg custard

FLAN MANZANA CON PURÉ DE FRESA, DE   apple flan with strawberry puree

FLAN NARANJA, DE   orange caramel custard

FLAN PEUADA, DE   pigs' feet mousse

FLAN UNIDAD   individual molded custard

FLAO   mint and cream cheese tart

FLAON   honey cheesecake with anisette liqueur and mint

FOIE GRAS FRANCÉS   French goose liver pâté

FONDAS ALCACHOFAS   artichoke bottoms

FONDOS DE ALCACHOFAS   artichoke bottoms

FONDOS DE ALCACHOFAS PATATAS   sauteed potatoes and artichoke bottoms

FONDUE BORGOÑA   cubes of beef that you cook at table using a long fork and dipping them into a pot of boiling oil

FRAMBUESA   raspberry

FRAMBUESA NATA   raspberries with cream

FRAMBUESA SILVESTRE   wild raspberry

FRANCESA   sauteed in butter

FREGINAT   white beans with fried pork liver

FRESA   strawberry

FRESA BORRACHA   strawberry with liquor
FRESA BOSQUE   wild strawberry
FRESA CON NATA   strawberry with cream
FRESA SILVESTRE   wild strawberry
FRESCO   fresh
FRESÓN   large strawberry
FRICADELAS   ground beef patties pan fried with sherry
   on fried French bread
FRICANDO   braised veal with wild mushrooms, pork,
   onion in tomato sauce
FRIJOLADA   bean stew with meats and vegetables
FRIJOLES   beans
FRIJOLES NEGROS   black beans
FRIJOLES REFRITOS   cooked beans, mashed and refried
FRÍO   cold
FRITE   pieces of a lamb yearling fried with paprika
FRITO   fried
FRITOS   fried appetizers
FRITURA   fry
FRITURA MIXTA   deep-fried meats, chicken, vegetables
   or fish
FRITURA MIXTA PESCADOS   deep-fried mixture of fish
FRUTA   fruit
FRUTA CON ALLIOLI   garlic mayonnaise with fruit
FRUTA ESCARCHADA   candied fruit
FRUTA MIXTA   assorted fruits
FRUTA SARTÉN, DE   dessert fritter
FRUTA SECA   dried fruit
FRUTA TIEMPO   fruit in season
FRUTAS DE MAR   seafoods
FUETE   sausage
FUNDADOR   wine distilled brandy

G

GALLETA   biscuit *or* cracker
GALLETA CON NATA   sandwich cookie with cream center

GALLINA   hen
GALLINA CON GARBANZOS   chicken stewed with chick-peas
GALLINA CON SALSA DE ALMENDRAS   stewed chicken in almond wine sauce
GALLINA GUINEA   guinea fowl
GALLINA PEPITORIA   chicken fricassee in saffron and garlic sauce
GALLO   cockerel rooster *or* black grouse
GAMBA   shrimp
GAMBA GRANDE   prawn
GAMBAS   large shrimp
GAMBAS AJILLOS, CON   shrimp with garlic mayonnaise sauce
GAMBAS, CÓCTEL DE   shrimp cocktail with mayonnaise sauce
GAMBAS DE LA BAYANA   prawns from the bay
GAMBAS GARBARDINA, CON   fried shrimp in a beer batter coating
GAMBAS JEREZ, CON   shrimp in dry sherry sauce
GAMBAS MAYONESA, CON   shrimp cocktail
GAMBAS SALSA PIPARRADA, CON   shrimp with tomato and pepper sauce
GAMBAS SALSA VERDE, CON   shrimp in green sauce
GAMBAS VILLEROY   boiled shrimp in a white bechamel sauce
GAMBONES   large prawns
GAMO   buck
GANSO   goose
GANSO CON ACEITUNAS   roast goose stuffed with veal, ham, garlic, onion
GARBANZOS   chick-peas
GARBANZOS CATALANA   chick-peas with tomato sauce
GARBANZOS REFRITOS   refried chick-peas
GAROM   anchovy-olive pâté
GARRAFA   carafe
GASEOSA   carbonated water

GATO FORMATGE   cheese cake

GAZPACHO   iced tomato and cucumber soup

GAZPACHO AJO BLANCO, CON   iced soup with almonds, garlic, oil, vinegar, grapes

GAZPACHO ANDALUZ   iced soup with tomatoes, green peppers, garlic, olive oil, wine vinegar, bread, ice water

GAZPACHO EXTREMEÑO   iced soup with garlic, green pepper, bread, eggs, olive oil, wine vinegar, ice water

GAZPACHO MADRILEÑO   iced soup with green peppers, tomatoes, garlic, olive oil, ice water, cucumber, bread cubes, wine vinegar, cumin seed

GAZPACHO MALAGÁN   iced soup with almonds, bread, wine vinegar, garlic, ice water, olive oil, white grapes

GAZPACHO SEVILLANO   iced soup with garlic, green pepper, onion, tomatoes, cucumber, olive oil, wine vinegar, ice water

GAZPACHUELO   fish soup with halibut, wine, clam juice, potatoes, vinegar

GELATINA AVE   cold, poached chicken stuffed with meat, rolled, covered with gelatin

GELATINA   gelatin

GELATINA CANYELLA   cinnamon ice cream with strawberry

GINEBRA   gin

GITANILLA   with garlic

GLASEADO   glazed

GOFIO   wheat flour, barley, corn or chick-peas, mixed with milk until a ball is formed

GORDO   rich or fatty food

GRACIAS   thank you

GRANADA   pomegranate

GRANADINA   eggplant and ground ham loaf

GRANADINAS   baked almond cinnamon cookies

GRAND MARNIER   orange flavored liqueur

GRANDE   large

GRANIZADO   shaved ice over strong, sweetened coffee or fruit syrup

GRATIN   cooked vegetables or pasta, baked in a casserole with butter, bread crumbs and grated cheese

GRATINADA CEBOLLA   onion soup with croutons and cheese

GRATINADO   gratineed

GRELOS   turnip greens

GRENADILLA   passion fruit

GRILLAJES   grilled dishes

GROSELLA   currant

GROSELLA ESPINOSA   gooseberry

GROSELLA NEGRA   black currant

GROSELLA ROJA   red currant

GUACAMOLE   pureed avocado, onion and seasonings

GUARNICIÓN   garnish

GUARNICIÓN DE VERDURAS   garnish of vegetables

GUAYABA   guava

GUINDA   sour cherry

GUINDILLA   chili pepper

GUISADO   stew

GUISADO ESPAÑOL   stew with beef, olive oil, onions

GUISANTES   green peas

GUISANTES AZÚCAR   peas glazed with butter and sugar

GUISANTES CATALANA   peas with raisins and pine nuts

GUISANTES CON TOCINO   peas with sauteed bacon

GUISANTES ESPAÑOLES   green peas sauteed with onion, carrot, ham

GUISANTES FRANCESES   peas with small onions, butter and lettuce

GUISANTES GRANADINAS, CON   cooked peas, artichoke hearts, sauteed onions, garlic, tomatoes and garnish of poached egg

GUISANTES MANTEQUILLA, CON   buttered peas

GUISANTES MENTA, CON   buttered peas with mint

GUISANTES PAISANOS   peas with small onions, butter and lettuce

GUISANTES REHOGADOS   peas sauteed in butter or oil

GUISANTES SALCHICHAS, CON   green peas with
   sausage, onion, tomato, garlic, mint
GUISANTES SALTEADOS CON JAMÓN   peas sauteed
   with ham
GUSANOS   sea snails
GUSTO   your taste or choice

H

HABAS   broad beans
HABAS ANDALUZA   lima beans with artichoke, cumin
   and eggs
HABAS CATALANA   broad beans with herbs, spices,
   mint, cinnamon
HABAS CON JAMÓN   lima beans or broad beans sauteed
   with wine and ham
HABICHUELAS   kidney beans
HABICHUELAS VERDES   string beans
HAMBURGUESA   hamburger
HAMBURGUESA LIONESA   hamburger with onion, pan
   fried with pan juices, wine and butter
HAMBURGUESA TIROLIENNE   pan fried hambuger
   with fried onion rings
HAYACA CENTRAL   cornmeal pancake with minced
   meat filling
HELADO   ice cream *or* any frozen dish
HELADO CHOCOLATE, DE   chocolate ice cream
HELADO CIRUELA PASA, DE   prune ice cream in orange
   liqueur sauce
HELADO HORNO, AL   Baked Alaska
HELADO JIJONA, CON   vanilla ice cream mixed with
   nougat candy
HELADO NATA, CON   ice cream with whipped cream
HELADO SEMIFRÍO   molded frozen dessert
HELADO TURRÓN, DE   vanilla ice cream with nougat
   candy mixed in
HELADO VAINILLA, DE   vanilla ice cream

HELADOS VARIADOS   various flavors of ice cream

HERVIDO   beef and vegetable stew

HIELO   ice

HIERBA   herb

HIERBAS FINAS   chopped mixture of herbs

HIGADILLOS   chicken livers

HIGADILLOS GELE OPORTO   chicken livers in port flavored aspic

HÍGADO   liver

HÍGADO CON AJO CABANIL   calves' liver sauteed in wine vinegar, garlic, paprika

HÍGADO CON CEBOLLAS   liver and onions

HÍGADO ENCEBOLLADO   liver sauteed with onions, peppers, wine

HÍGADO INGLÉS   thin slices of liver, coated in flour, fried in butter

HÍGADO LIONÉS   liver fried in butter with onions and a sauce from pan juices

HÍGADO PIMENTOS, CON   calves' liver pan fried in onions and peppers

HIGO   fig

HINOJO   fennel, a licorice tasting vegetable like celery

HOJALDRA   puff pastry used for dessert or with fillings of meat and fish

HOJAS DE PARRA RELLENAS   meat stuffed grape leaves stewed in tomato sauce

HOLANDESA   Hollandaise sauce, made with lemon juice flavored egg yolks and butter

HONGO   mushroom

HORCHATA   almond or coconut flavored soft drink served cold

HORCHATA DE ALMENDRA   drink made of ground almonds

HORNO   baked

HORTALIZA   greens

HUACHINANGO   red snapper

HUESO   bone

HUEVAS ALIÑADAS   seasoned fish roe
HUEVAS NIEVE, CON   egg shaped meringue, poached in vanilla flavored boiling milk, served with custard sauce
HUEVO ESCALFADO   soup with poached egg
HUEVOS   eggs; also see TORTILLA
HUEVOS A SU GUSTO   eggs prepared to your choice
HUEVOS ALCACHOFAS, CON   eggs with artichoke hearts
HUEVOS ANCHOAS, CON   eggs with anchovies
HUEVOS ATÚN, CON   eggs with tuna fish
HUEVOS BACALAO, CON   eggs with dried codfish
HUEVOS BESAMEL, CON   eggs with white sauce of butter, flour and milk; Bechamel sauce
HUEVOS BUTIFARRA, CON   eggs with sausage
HUEVOS CAZUELA, EN   eggs baked in a casserole
HUEVOS CEBOLLA, CON   eggs with onion
HUEVOS CHAMPIÑONES, CON   eggs with mushrooms
HUEVOS CHORIZO, CON   eggs with paprika flavored sausage
HUEVOS COCIDOS   boiled eggs
HUEVOS COCOTTE   shirred eggs
HUEVOS CON ALLIOLI   eggs with garlic mayonnaise
HUEVOS CREMA, CON   eggs with cream sauce
HUEVOS CUBANOS   fried eggs on rice, topped with fried bananas and tomato sauce
HUEVOS DEL MESÓN   special restaurant preparation of eggs
HUEVOS DUROS   hard cooked eggs
HUEVOS ESCALFADOS   shirred eggs
HUEVOS ESCALFADOS BENEDICTINOS   poached eggs on ham covered toast with Hollandaise sauce or a cream sauce
HUEVOS ESCALFADOS CON CREMA   eggs poached in cream
HUEVOS ESPAÑOLES   eggs stuffed with tomatoes, with cheese sauce
HUEVOS ESPÁRRAGOS, CON   eggs with asparagus
HUEVOS ESPEJO   eggs coated with cream and cooked

HUEVOS ESPINACAS, CON   eggs with spinach

HUEVOS FLAMENCOS   eggs on a bed of tomatoes, chorizo, ham, green beans, fried potatoes, asparagus, red pepper and peas, in small pieces, put in the oven

HUEVOS FLORENTINOS   eggs with spinach and grated cheese or cheese sauce

HUEVOS FRITOS   fried eggs

HUEVOS FRITOS AMERICANOS   fried eggs, bacon, ham and tomato

HUEVOS FRITOS CON AJILLO   eggs fried in olive oil with garlic and paprika

HUEVOS FRITOS ESPAÑOLES   eggs fried in olive oil served with sausage, potatoes, croutons

HUEVOS FRITOS HUERTANOS   fried eggs with mixed vegetables

HUEVOS FRITOS SEVILLANOS   fried eggs with ham, anchovy stuffed olives, sausage; *or* nests of tomatoes, onion, garlic and ham with fried egg placed in middle

HUEVOS GELATINA, CON   eggs in aspic

HUEVOS GRAN DUQUESA   poached eggs on fried bread with truffle, cheese sauce and grated cheese, asparagus, crayfish tails, oven-browned

HUEVOS GRATINADOS   eggs covered with sauce, bread crumbs, grated cheese and then browned

HUEVOS GUISADOS   eggs fried in olive oil

HUEVOS GUISANTES, CON   eggs with peas

HUEVOS HIGADILLOS DE POLLO, CON   eggs with chicken livers

HUEVOS HOLANDESES   eggs with cream sauce of egg yolks, butter and lemon juice

HUEVOS HORNO, AL   baked eggs

HUEVOS LANGOSTINOS   eggs with prawns

HUEVOS LONGANIZA, CON   eggs with sausage

HUEVOS MADRILEÑOS   eggs baked with sausage, tomatoes, grated cheese

HUEVOS MAGRA CABALLO   slice of fried ham topped with a fried egg

HUEVOS MANTUA   eggs with sauce made using
  crayfish stock
HUEVOS MARISCOS, CON   eggs with seafood
HUEVOS MAYONESA   hard -boiled eggs with mayonnaise
HUEVOS MEYERBEER   eggs with lamb kidney and
  truffle sauce
HUEVOS MIGAS, CON   scrambled eggs with fried bread
  croutons
HUEVOS MOLDEADOS   eggs cooked in a mold
HUEVOS MORCILLA, CON   eggs with blood sausage
HUEVOS MORNAY   eggs with white cream sauce and
  grated cheese
HUEVOS NATURALES   plain eggs
HUEVOS NIDO, EN   egg yolk placed in roll, fried and
  covered with egg white
HUEVOS PARMESANOS   eggs with grated Parmesan
  cheese
HUEVOS PASADOS POR AGUA   soft-boiled eggs
HUEVOS PATATAS, CON   eggs with potatoes
HUEVOS PICADILLOS CON CHAMPIÑONES   eggs
  baked on top of chopped mushrooms
HUEVOS PIPERADOS VASCOS   scrambled eggs with bell
  peppers, tomatoes, onions and fried ham
HUEVOS PISTO   eggs with cooked vegetables
HUEVOS RELLENOS CON GAMBAS   hard-boiled eggs
  stuffed with shrimp
HUEVOS RELLENOS CON SALMÓN   salmon stuffed
  hard-boiled eggs
HUEVOS REVUELTOS   scrambled eggs; also see
  TORTILLAS
HUEVOS RUSOS FRÍOS   cold, stuffed hard-boiled egg
  halves with mayonnaise
HUEVOS SALMORREJO   eggs baked in olive oil, garlic,
  onion, with ham, pork loin, sausage and asparagus
  spears
HUEVOS TOCINO, CON   bacon and eggs
HUMITA   corn, tomatoes, green peppers, onion, cheese

I

IGLESIA   underdone; boiled; with boiled vegetables

ISCATÓN   marinated liver with red wine sauce

J

JABALÍ   wild boar

JABALÍ, CABEZA DE   de-boned boar's head with stuffing containing pistachio nuts

JABALÍ EN ADOBO, CHULETAS DE   wild boar chops marinated, grilled or broiled with spicy sauce

JABALÍ, LOMO DE   saddle of boar

JABALÍ, PERNIL DE   haunch of boar

JALEA   jellied

JAMÓN   ham, mostly air-dried and cured

JAMÓN AGUADILLA   roast fresh ham

JAMÓN AÑEJO CON PEPINILLOS   aged ham with pickles

JAMÓN BIGARADE   ham boiled, baked, served in Madeira wine sauce with orange juice

JAMÓN CANUTILLOS, CON   slices of ham rolled and filled

JAMÓN COCIDO   boiled ham

JAMÓN CRUDO   cold, boiled ham

JAMÓN DULCE   ham boiled and served cold

JAMÓN GALLEGO   thinly sliced smoked ham

JAMÓN HUEVO HILADO, CON   boiled ham with egg and sugar mixture coating

JAMÓN, LONCHAS DE   thin slices of ham

JAMÓN MELÓN, Y   ham and melon

JAMÓN OPORTO, CON   ham boiled, baked in a port wine butter sauce

JAMÓN PEPINILLOS, CON   cold boiled ham with pickles

JAMÓN SERRANO   dried ham

JAMÓN TACOS, EN   diced ham

JAMÓN VARIANTE   sliced ham with various garnishes

JAMÓN VIRUTAS   thin slices of ham

JAMÓN YORK   boiled ham

JARDINERA   with carrots, peas and mixed vegetables

JARRETE   veal *or* lamb shank

JENGIBRE   ginger

JEREZ   sherry

JUDÍAS   beans

JUDÍAS BLANCAS   white beans

JUDÍAS ESPAÑOLAS   string beans cooked in sauce of
    tomato, onion, garlic flavored olive oil

JUDÍAS OREJA PIE CERDO   stew of white beans, pig's
    ears and feet in onion, garlic, tomato gravy

JUDÍAS PINTAS   pinto beans

JUDÍAS ROJAS   red *or* kidney beans

JUDÍAS VERDES   string beans

JUDÍAS VERDES CON AJO   green beans with butter and
    garlic

JUDÍAS VERDES CON BARCENA   green beans sauteed
    with olive oil and ham

JUDÍAS VERDES CON SALSA DE TOMATE   green beans
    in tomato sauce

JUGO   juice

JUGO NARANJA, DE   orange juice

JUGO PIÑA, DE   pineapple juice

JUGO TOMATE, DE   tomato juice

JUGO TORONJA, DE   grapefruit juice

JULIANNA   shredded vegetables

JUREL   kind of mackerel

K

KIRSCH   white cherry liquor

KOKOTXAS   hake fish

L

LA ROSTA   thick bread slices toasted with garlic spread
    then dipped in hot olive oil

LACÓN   pork shoulder

LACÓN CURADO   salted pork

LACÓN GRELOS   boiled pork hocks, potatoes, sausage, Swiss chard

LAMPREA   sea or fresh water fish that looks like an eel

LAMPREA BORDELESA   fresh water fish with leeks and wine

LANGOSTA   lobster

LANGOSTA AJO ARRIERO, CON   lobster, onion, garlic, wine, vinegar

LANGOSTA AMERICANA   boiled pieces of lobster with sauce of tomatoes, onions, white wine, paprika or mild red pepper, oven-browned

LANGOSTA CARDINAL   pieces of boiled lobster with truffle slices on mushrooms, with grated cheese, oven browned, with tomato wine sauce

LANGOSTA CATALANA   lobster braised in white wine, onion and fish broth, with almond paste

LANGOSTA COSTA BRAVA, DE   lobster tails, mushroom, ham, scallion, wine

LANGOSTA HERVIDA   boiled lobster

LANGOSTA NEWBURG   lobster sauteed in thick white sauce, cream and wine

LANGOSTA POBRE   poor man's lobster, made from white fish, garlic, carrots, olive oil

LANGOSTA POLLO, Y   chicken and lobster braised with onion and tomato, with paste of garlic, almonds, chestnuts, chicken liver

LANGOSTA THERMIDOR   lobster braised in sherry cream sauce, mustard flavored fish stock, with cheese and oven browned

LANGOSTINOS   shellfish similar to shrimp; also see GAMBAS

LANGOSTINOS CLAVO, CON   boiled large shrimp in wine, pepper, clove, peppercorn sauce

LANGOSTINOS GRAN MESÓN   prawns in garlic onion sauce

LANGOSTINOS PARRILLA, A LA   shrimp grilled on a
steel plate, basted with olive oil
LASAÑA   a wide flat noodle
LASAÑA HORNO   lasagne with alternating layers of
mozzarella, ricotta cheese, meat-tomato sauce, baked
LASAÑA VERDE   green lasagna made with spinach dough
LAUREL   bay leaf
LAVAR   to wash
LECHAL   milk fed veal
LECHE   milk
LECHE DULCE   sweet, thick cream of boiled milk
LECHE FRITA   fried custard squares
LECHE FRITA CON ANÍS   fried milk custard with flamed
anisette liqueur
LECHE MERENGADA   cinnamon flavored ice milk
LECHECILLAS   sweetbreads
LECHÓN   suckling pig
LECHUGA   lettuce
LECHUGA BRASEADA CON JUGO   braised lettuce
LEGUMBRE   vegetable
LEGUMBRES RELLENAS   stuffed vegetables
LENGUA   tongue
LENGUA GELATINA, CON   tongue in aspic
LENGUA PORTUGUESA   tongue braised in tomato,
onion, oil
LENGUA SEVILLANA   tongue with green olives, pota-
toes, red peppers
LENGUADO   sole, a flounder-like fish
LENGUADO ALBARINO   filet of sole in wine mushroom
sauce
LENGUADO ALMENDRAS, CON   filet of sole fried in
butter with sliced almonds and lemons
LENGUADO AURORA   poached filets with creamy
sauce, tomato puree added
LENGUADO CAFÉ PARÍS, DE   filet of sole poached in
stock with truffles, mushrooms, asparagus tips, prawns
in creamy lobster sauce

LENGUADO CHAMPAGNE, EN   filet of sole poached in champagne

LENGUADO COLBERT, CON   filet of sole breaded, deep-fried, stuffed with lemon butter

LENGUADO DELICIAS   filets of sole, poached, covered with creamy sauce

LENGUADO DONOSTIARRA, CON   filets immered in butter and bouillon under a tomato sauce

LENGUADO ERMITAÑO   filets stuffed with crumbs, eggs, herbs, shallots, braised, served with creamy sauce

LENGUADO ESCORIAL   filet of sole oven poached in fish stock, covered with pink wine sauce

LENGUADO, FILETES DE   filets of sole, flat sea fish

LENGUADO FRITO   fried filet of sole with vegetables

LENGUADO GOUGONS   strips of filets, floured and deep-fried

LENGUADO INGLÉS   filet of sole coated with beaten egg and bread crumbs and deep-fried

LENGUADO, LAZOS DE   strips of filets, deep-fried

LENGUADO LIMÓN, CON   filet of flounder in lemon wine sauce

LENGUADO MARGUERITE   filet of sole poached in wine with white sauce

LENGUADO MARGUERY   filet of sole poached in fish stock and wine, with creamy wine sauce, oven browned

LENGUADO MAYONESA VERDE, CON   fish filet with green mayonnaise sauce

LENGUADO MEUNIERE   whole sole floured, fried in butter

LENGUADO MILANESA, A LA   filet of sole egg coated, breaded with crumbs and grated Parmesan cheese, then fried

LENGUADO MOLINERA   filets fried in butter on butter fried sliced mushrooms

LENGUADO MUJER   filet of sole poached in white wine on mushrooms, oven browned

LENGUADO MURAT   strips of fried sole mixed with diced potato and artichoke hearts

LENGUADO NARANJA, CON   filet of sole garnished
  with orange
LENGUADO NORMANDA   filet of sole poached in fish
  stock covered with mushrooms, mussels and shrimp,
  covered with creamy sauce and oven browned
LENGUADO ORLI   filets breaded, deep-fried, served
  with lemon slices
LENGUADO OTELLO   filets on baked potatoes, creamed
  chopped shrimp, browned with creamy cheese sauce
LENGUADO PIÑONES, CON   fish filet with pine nuts
  and beef sauce
LENGUADO POPIETAS, CON   poached filets with
  creamy sauce
LENGUADO RELLENO   stuffed sole
LENGUADO ROMANO   poached filets on macaroni with
  grated Parmesan, anchovies, covered with white sauce
  and oven browned
LENGUADO SALSA DE NUECES, CON   sole filets in nut
  sauce
LENGUADO TÍO PEPE   filet of sole poached in stock and
  sherry, covered with creamy sauce
LENGUAS DE GATO   wafer thin crisp cookies served
  with ice cream or custard
LENTEJAS   lentils
LIBRE   vacant
LICOR   liqueur
LIEBRE   hare
LIEBRE CIVET   stew of hare with onions and mushrooms
LIEBRE ESTOFADA   jugged hare
LIEBRE FABES   hare braised and stewed with broad beans
LIMA   lime
LIMÓN   lemon
LIMONADA   lemonade
LIMONADA MADRILEÑA   red wine, lemon juice, peach
  and lemon wedges and water
LISTA DE PLATOS   menu
LISTA DE VINOS   wine list

LIVIANO   light
LLAGOSTA   spiny lobster
LLAGOSTÍN   prawn
LLAMA   flamed with brandy
LLAMANTO   lobster
LLAME   knock
LLAME AL TIMBRE   ring
LLAMINADURE   pastry, dessert, sweet
LLAUNA   baking dish
LLENTIE   lentil
LLOBARRO   sea bass
LLOBARRO FORN   baked sea bass
LLOM   loin of pork
LLUC   hake fish
LOBARRO   bass
LOCRO   corn soup stew of South America
LOMBARDA   red cabbage
LOMBARDA RELLENA   baked sausage stuffed red
   cabbage
LOMO   loin, usually pork
LOMO ADOBADO   pork loin marinated and roasted with
   lard and potatoes
LOMO CERDO ARAGONÉS, DE   loin of pork with
   onions and white wine
LOMO CERDO ESCALIBADO, DE   roast pork with egg-
   plant, red and green peppers
LOMO CERDO ZARAGOZANO, DE   pork chops with
   tomato sauce and black olives
LOMO, CINTA DE   boned loin of pork
LOMO EMBUCHADO   stuffed loin
LOMO MONTADITO   pork loin on a slice of bread
LOMO PUERCO CON PIMIENTOS VERMELHOS DUCES,
   DE   pork loin with sweet red peppers
LOMO RELLENO SALCHICHA   sausage wrapped in
   pork slices, sauteed with onion, garlic, wine
LONCHAS   cut in thin slices
LONGANIZA   sausage

LONJA   slice of meat

LUBINA   sea bass

LUBINA ALBUFERA   bass baked in garlic almond sauce

LUBINA CORTA CON CALDO   bass poached in a
vegetable bouillon

LUBINA HINOJO, CON   bass marinated in oil, lemon
juice and fennel, then grilled

LUBINA NARANJA, CON   fish fried, served with orange
sections and orange flavored sauce

LUBINA SALSA TÁRTARA, CON   bass poached with
tartar sauce

LUBINA SANTURCE   bass lightly fried, then oven baked
with vinegar and fried minced garlic

LUBINA SUPREME VERÓNICA   filets poached in fish
stock with orange liqueur, covered with a sauce, oven
browned

LUBINA VINO BLANCO, CON   bass poached in white
wine

LUBRICANTE   lobster with claws

LUCIO   pike

M

MACARRONES   macaroni

MACEDONIA DE FRUTA   fruit salad

MADEJAS   lamb intestines wrapped around garlic and
roasted

MADRILEÑA   with sausage, tomatoes and paprika

MADUIXA   strawberry

MAGANOS   squid

MAGRAS   thick slice of lean ham fried in lard or butter,
with tomatoes and vegetables

MAGRAS CON TOMATE   slices of slightly fried ham
dipped in tomato sauce

MAGRAS ESTILO ARAGÓN   cured ham in tomato sauce

MAÎTRE D'HÔTEL SALSA   butter creamed with lemon
juice

MAÍZ   corn
MÁLAGA   dessert wine
MALLORQUINA   highly seasoned fish and shellfish
MANCHEGO   Spanish cheese
MANDARINA   mandarin orange
MANDONGUILLE   meatball
MANGO   tropical fruit
MANÍ   peanut
MANITAS   lamb's feet
MANJAR BLANCO   almond-milk pudding
MANOS   pig's feet
MANOS DE CERDO RELLENAS   stuffed pigs' feet
MANTECA NEGRA   browned butter
MANTECADA   sweet dough baked and sprinkled with
   sugar and cinnamon
MANTECADAS ASTORGA   cinnamon muffins
MANTECADO   ice cream with frozen whipped cream
   texture; French ice cream
MANTECADOS   cookies
MANTEQUILLA   butter
MANTEQUILLA FUNDIDA   melted butter
MANZANA   apple
MANZANA ASADA   baked apple
MANZANA DULCE   apple in honey
MANZANILLA   dry white wine
MAR   fish and seafood
MARGARITA   tequila with lime juice
MARINERA   with mussels, onions, tomatoes
MARISCADA   mixed seafood grill
MARISCADA MARINERA   baked clams, mussels and
   other shellfish
MARISCADA PLANCHA, A LA   shellfish grilled over
   charcoal
MARISCOS   shellfish
MARISCOS COSTA BRAVA   shellfish in spiced tomato sauce
MARISCOS FIDEUA   noodles with fish, shrimp, toma-
   toes, fish broth

MARMITKO   soup of tuna, tomato, onion, brandy, potatoes, green pepper

MARQUESITAS   chocolate confections made with chopped almonds, sugar and egg yolk

MASA SOBADA   Portuguese sweet bread

MASITAS   cupcakes

MATAMBRE   beef rolled and stuffed with vegetables

MAYONESA   mayonnaise

MAZAGRÁN   lemon flavored iced coffee

MAZAPÁN   almond paste

MAZAPÁN DE TOLEDO   paste of ground almonds, sugar and egg whites

MEDIA BOTELLA   half bottle

MEDIAS NOCHES   small buns often used for tea sandwiches or snacks

MEJILLONES   mussels marinated in oil, vinegar, capers, onion

MEJILLONES AMERICANOS   poached mussels with tomato sauce, simmered in oven

MEJILLONES BERCY   mussels poached in white wine, served with sauce of reduced poaching liquor

MEJILLONES CON SALSA VERDE   mussels in wine, oil, onion, garlic sauce

MEJILLONES GRATINADOS   baked mussels and mushrooms

MEJILLONES MARINEROS   mussels simmered in white wine, served in this steaming liquor

MEJILLONES POULETTE   mussels poached on half-shell with creamy stock mushroom sauce

MEJILLONES RELLENOS   mussels poached on half-shell with garlic butter

MEJORANA   marjoram

MEL I MATO   patty of cottage cheese with honey and roasted hazelnuts

MELAZA   molasses

MELBA   fruits poached in syrup with vanilla ice cream and raspberry sauce

MELINDRES YEPES   almond marzipan candies
MELOCOTÓN   peach
MELOCOTÓN MELBA   peach poached in syrup with
   vanilla ice cream and raspberry sauce
MELÓN   melon
MELÓN JAMÓN, CON   melon with raw cured ham
MELÓN MIEL, CON   honey melon
MELÓN OPORTO   melon flavored with port wine
MEMBRILLO   quince jelly dessert
MEMBRILLO CON QUESO   quince jelly slice eaten with
   cheese
MENESTRA   green vegetable soup
MENESTRA ACELGAS, CON   Swiss chard and potato
   casserole with egg crust
MENESTRA LEGUMBRES, CON   mixed vegetable
   casserole
MENESTRA POLLO, CON   chicken vegetable soup
MENESTRA RIOJANA, CON   baked vegetable casserole
MENESTRA VERDURAS, CON   mixed sauteed vegetables
MENESTRONE   vegetable soup
MENTA   mint
MENÚ DEL DÍA   set menu
MENÚ TURÍSTICO   tourist menu
MENUDILLOS   giblets
MENUDILLOS DE GALLINA   chicken giblets; livers,
   hearts, gizzards, kidneys
MENUDILLOS DE POLLO   cold poultry
MERENGUE   meringue
MERIENDA   late afternoon meal
MERLUZA   hake, like codfish
MERLUZA AMERICANA   hake breaded and pan fried in
   sauce of oil, wine, onions, cheese
MERLUZA ANZUELO, CON   hake fritters
MERLUZA BATELERA   hake poached with puree of
   mussels and cream
MERLUZA BILBAÍNA   hake dipped in egg, fried in deep
   fat

MERLUZA BLANCA   hake poached with sauce on the side or oil and vinegar

MERLUZA CATALANA   braised hake

MERLUZA, COLA DE   tail of hake

MERLUZA CON AJILLO   poached hake with garlic flavored mayonnaise

MERLUZA COSQUERA   hake lightly fried in olive oil with garlic, wine, sauteed clams

MERLUZA, EMPAREDADOS DE   fried hake and ham slices

MERLUZA CECILIA, FILETE DE   hake pan fried in butter with asparagus tips

MERLUZA GALLEGA   baked fish with potato, paprika, onion, clove

MERLUZA GRANADINA   hake with fried garlic, peppers, onions, tomatoes, wine, simmered in oven

MERLUZA HERVIDA   hake poached in sauce

MERLUZA HORNO, AL   baked hake with potatoes and tomato sauce

MERLUZA JAIZKIBEL   cod or hake in rich wine sauce

MERLUZA KOSKERA   hake sauteed with clams, olive oil, garlic, wine, asparagus and green peas

MERLUZA MADRILEÑA   codfish stuffed with ham, cheese, bread crumbs battered and fried

MERLUZA MARINERA   poached hake filets with tomato and almond sauce

MERLUZA PAPEL CON JAMÓN, EN   hake marinated with slices of ham, sealed in oiled paper and oven baked

MERLUZA PLANCHA, A LA   hake grilled on a steel plate

MERLUZA PRIMAVERA   poached filets of cod or hake with green cream sauce

MERLUZA, PUDÍN DE   pudding of mashed hake, onion, tomato paste, oil, cooked, chilled and covered with mayonnaise

MERLUZA REBOZADA   battered and deep-fried hake

MERLUZA RIOJANA   hake with a tomato puree, peppers and garlic olive oil

MERLUZA ROMANA   battered and deep-fried hake
MERLUZA ROMESCA   hake in peppery sauce
MERLUZA SALSA VERDE, CON   hake with garlic,
   clams, green peas, asparagus
MERLUZA SIDRA, CON   fish in cider with clams, onion,
   potatoes, garlic
MERLUZA TROPICAL   hake sauteed and baked with
   bananas, onion, raisins, almonds, pineapple and sherry
MERLUZA VASCA   slices of hake simmered in oil with
   garlic, then put in earthenware casserole with sauce of
   fish stock, garlic and parsley and simmered in oven
MERMELADA   jam
MERMELADA DE NARANJA   marmelade, orange jam
MERO   halibut, pollack or sea bass
MERO BILBAÍNA   baked halibut with peppers
MERO BORGOÑONA   halibut poached in red wine
MERO CANTÁBRICO   halibut poached with sauce from
   onions, garlic, potato, parsley, olive oil and vinegar
MERO HORNO, AL   halibut baked with potatoes and
   onion
MERO MARINERO   halibut fried in oil, simmered with
   onion, bell pepper and garlic
MERO PLANCHA, A LA   halibut grilled on a steel plate
MERO SALSA VERDE, CON   pollock in green sauce
MESERA   waitress
MESERO   waiter
MESÓN   the restaurant
MEZCLADO   mixed
MICHIRONES   lima beans *or* broad beans; also see
   HABAS
MICHIRONES PICANTICOS   spicy lima beans with sau-
   sage and chili pepper
MIEL   honey
MIGAS   bread soaked in water, fried with bacon and dry
   peppers
MIL HOJAS CREMA   pastry layered with custard and
   frosted on top

MILANESA   baked with cheese

MINUTA   menu

MIRABEL   yellow plum

MIXTO   mixed

MIXTO GRILL   mixed grilled meat

MOJE MANCHEGO   cold broth with black olives

MOJETE   potatoes sauteed with garlic, paprika, tomato and bay leaf, with poached egg added

MOJO   dressing made with oil, vinegar, garlic, salt, spices; for color: paprika for red, piquant peppers for picon, coriander for green

MOKA   mocha coffee

MOLE GUAJALOTE   turkey dish of Mexico, with garlic, tortillas, onion, tomatoes, chocolate

MOLE POBLANO   chicken with sauce of chili peppers and chocolate

MOLINERA   fish floured and pan fried in butter

MOLLEJA   gizzard

MOLLEJAS   sweetbreads

MOLLEJAS CAZADORA   sweetbreads braised in wine, mushrooms, shallots, tomato paste

MOLLEJAS JEREZ, CON   sweetbreads sauteed and served in sauce of pan juices and sherry

MOLLEJAS PROVENZALE   fried slices of sweetbreads with tomato sauce, anchovies, wine and oil

MOLLEJAS REBOZO, DE   sweetbreads slices coated in batter and deep fried

MOLLEJAS VINO MADEIRA   sweetbreads with Madeira sauce, pan juices and mushrooms

MOLUSCO   snail, mussel, clam

MONDONGO   thick vegetable soup or stew

MONJET   black-eyed pea

MONJETAS   dried white beans

MONTILLA   dessert wine

MORA   mulberry

MORCILLA   mild blood sausage

MORCILLO   veal shank

MORILLA   morel mushroom
MORNAY   creamy cheese sauce
MOROS CRISTIANOS   rice, black beans, ham, garlic, green peppers
MORRO   pig snout
MORRO ANDALUZ   pig snout stewed in sauce of mint, beans, onion, tomato, pimento, ham and chorizo
MORTERUELO   pork liver, giblets, game and a variety of spices
MORUNA   pork in barbecue sauce
MOSCATEL   muscatel
MOSTACHONES   small cakes for dipping in coffee or hot chocolate
MOSTAZA   mustard
MOUSSE DE CHOCOLATE   frothy chocolate pudding dessert
MOUSSE FETGE POLLASTRE   chicken liver mousse
MOUSSELINE (SALSA)   Hollandaise sauce with added whipped cream
MOZO   youth
MUJOL   mullet
MUJOL HUEVAS   mullet roe, pan fried in butter
MUSCO GRATINATS   gratineed mussel
MUSLO DE CONEJO   roasted rabbit thigh
MUY SECO   very dry

N

NABOS   turnips
NARANJA   orange
NARANJADA   orangeade
NATA   cream
NATA BATIDA   whipped cream
NATA MONTADA   whipped cream
NATILLAS   custard
NATILLAS BIZCOCHO, CON   custard over ladyfinger
NATILLAS ESPAÑOLAS   custard over sweet biscuit

NATILLAS LIMÓN, DE lemon cream
NATILLAS NUECES, CON soft milk custard with walnuts
NATURAL plain
NAVAJAS razor fish
NAVIZA young turnip greens
NECORAS crab
NEULE rolled cookie
NICALOS wild mushroom
NÍSPERO tart fruit that grows wild
NO-ALCOHÓLICO non-alcoholic
NOPALES edible cactus
NOPALITO cactus leaf with salad dressing
ÑOQUIS dumplings of potatoes, boiled with a sauce of
 butter and grated cheese, oven browned
ÑOQUIS PARISINA flour dumplings with cheese sauce,
 oven browned
NOUILLES fresh noodles
NOUILLES VERDES green noodles made with cooked
 spinach in the raw dough
NUECES nuts
NUEZ MOSCADA nutmeg

O

OCA goose
OCA CON PERAS baby roast goose with pine nuts,
 raisins, pears, wine, with pears caramelized after
 cooking
OCUPADO engaged, occupied
OLIAIGUA olive oil soup
OLIAIGUA TOMATES olive oil soup with tomatoes
OLIVES olives
OLLA stew *or* soup
OLLA DE ESCUDELLA CON CARNE soup with boiled
 meats and vegetables
OLLA GITANA vegetable stew
OLLA PESCADOS seafood stew

OLLA PODRIDA   stew of ham, chick-peas, cabbage, leeks, tomatoes, chorizo

OLLITA   pot used for stew; stew

OLOROSO   sweet, dark sherry

OMELETTE ALASKA   dessert with ice cream center covered with meringue, oven browned and flamed with brandy

OMELETTE SURPRISE   Baked Alaska

OPORTO   port

OSSO BUCCO   veal shank braised in onion, garlic, tomato

OSTIONES   small shellfish, like oysters

OSTRAS   oysters

OSTRAS, 1/2 DOCENA DE   half a dozen oysters

OSTRAS MORNAY   poached oysters with white cheese sauce and oven browned

OUS   eggs; also see HUEVOS

OVAS MOLES   egg yolk icing

OVEJA   ewe

P

PA TOMAQUET   tomato bread

PABELLÓN CRIOLLO   beef in tomato sauce with beans, rice and bananas

PAELLA   stew of pork, rice, chicken, clams, shrimp

PAELLA ALICANTINA   rice, chicken and rabbit stew

PAELLA ARAGONESA   stew of rabbit, pork, squid, tomato, onion, peas, bell pepper, garlic and saffron

PAELLA BARCELONESA   stew of rice, chicken, chicken liver, squid, fish, onion, tomatoes, garlic, green pepper, mussels, shrimp, olive oil, sausage, peas, saffron, artichokes

PAELLA CATALANA   stew of rice, sausages, pork, squid, tomatoes, peppers and peas

PAELLA CODORNICES Y SETAS, CON   stew with rice, rabbit, pork, quail, tomato, beans, onions, mushrooms, garlic, pork ribs

PAELLA HUERTANA MURCIA   stew with rice, green beans, peas, lima beans, tomato, artichoke hearts

PAELLA MARINERA   stew of rice with fish, shellfish and meat

PAELLA MARISCOS CON POLLO, DE   stew with seafood and chicken

PAELLA MARISCOS, DE   rice and shellfish stew

PAELLA MILANESA   stew of rice in broth with sauteed onion, wine and saffron

PAELLA PARELLADA   stew of rice containing chicken, meat, sausage, fish, seafood, onions, garlic, tomato and peas

PAELLA VALENCIANA   stew with rice, chicken, pimentos, shellfish and saffron

PALITOS   toothpicks with bits of delicacies, such as pickled vegetables, ham, cheese, smoked fish

PALMITO   palm heart

PALOMA   dove

PALOMINO   pigeon

PALTA   avocado

PAMBOLI TOMATIGA   tomato bread

PAN   bread

PAN CANDEAL   country style bread, slightly sour

PAN CEBADO   strong flavored corn and barley bread

PAN GALLEGO DE CENTENO   round rye bread

PAN MUNICIÓN   chocolate custard cake with chocolate sauce

PAN PUEBLO, DE   white bread loaf

PAN QUEMADO   sweet bread with baked egg white topping

PAN SANTA TERESA   French toast

PAN TOSTADO   toasted bread

PANACHE   mixed

PANACHE LEGUMBRES, DE   variety of fresh vegetables sauteed together

PANACHE VERDURAS, DE   mixed sauteed vegetables

PANECILLO   French roll

PANELLET   marzipan cookie

PANELLETS   Catalán almond cookies

PAPAS   South American potatoes

PAPAS ARRUGAS, CON   potatoes baked in their jackets

PAPAS FRITAS   South American fried potatoes

PAPAS HUANCAINA   potatoes, cheese and green peppers

PAPAYA   a tropical fruit

PAPOS ANJO   egg cakes in syrup

PARFAIT   ice cream mixed with egg yolks, cooked and
cooled, whipped cream and flavorings added, then
chilled in a mold

PARMESANA   Parmesan cheese

PARRILLA   grilled over an open fire

PARRILLA DE GERONA   veal steak

PARRILLA MIXTA   mixed grill

PARRILLADA INGLESA   mixed grill

PARRILLADA MARISCOS   broiled seafoods or fish

PARRILLADA MIXTA   mixed grill

PASADO   done, cooked

PASAS   raisins

PASAS Y PIÑONES   raisins and pine nuts

PASTA DE HÍGADO DE GANSO   goose liver pâté

PASTA HOJALDRADA   filled puff pastry

PASTA ITALIANA   spaghetti

PASTAS   pastry

PASTAS BAVARAS   spatzle, small dumplings made of
dough

PASTEL   baked puff pastry pie sometimes with sausage,
ham, peppers and onion or a meat loaf

PASTEL CHOCLO   corn, chopped beef, chicken, raisins
and olives

PASTEL CIERVA   pie made with veal, chorizo, hard egg,
brains and minced meat in pastry and baked

PASTEL HELADO   liquor soaked sponge cake with ice
cream

PASTEL HOJALDRADO   puff pastry *or* cream puff

PASTEL MANZANA, DE   apple-mint crisp

PASTEL MURCIANO   baked veal, ham, pepper, tomato pie

PASTEL NATA Y CREMA, CON   pastry with whipped cream and custard

PASTEL NUECES, CON   pastry with chopped nuts

PASTEL PERDIZ   partridge pâté

PASTEL PUERROS Y GAMBAS, CON   shrimp and leek pâté

PASTEL SUIZO   individual pastries sprinkled with sugar

PASTEL YEMA HELADO   pastry made with egg-yolk and sugar cream filling, frozen

PASTELERÍA   pastry *or* pastry shop

PASTELERÍA FINA   delicate pastry

PASTELES   cakes

PASTELES FRUTAS, DE   fruit tarts

PASTELES HIGOS, CON   baked puff pastry with fig and candied squash filling

PASTELILLO   little tart

PASTELITOS   small cakes

PASTELS NATA   custard tarts

PASTITAS   soup dumplings

PASTORA   lamb and vegetable stew

PATA   foot

PATA DE CERDO COCIDA   pickled pork

PATAS DE CERDO   pigs' feet

PATAS DE CERDO DUROC   poached pigs' feet with brown beef sauce

PATAS DE CERDO EN BRETONA   stewed pigs' feet in tomato sauce with white beans

PATATA FRITA   deep-fried potato patty

PATATAS   potatoes

PATATAS ASADAS   baked potatoes

PATATAS COCIDAS   boiled potatoes

PATATAS FRITAS   French fried potatoes

PATATAS SALSA VERDE, CON   potatoes in green parsley sauce

PATATAS SALTEADAS   fried potatoes

PATATE ALLIOLI   potato with olive oil and garlic

PATATE CATALANA   stuffed potato

PATATE RABASSOLE   potato with mushroom
PATATES   potatoes
PATATES ASADOS   roasted potatoes
PATATES ASADOS RELLENOS   stuffed baked potatoes
    with ham
PATATES BRAVOS   potato cubes in thick spicy tomato
    pepper sauce
PATATES CHORIZO, CON   potato cubes with sausage
    and bacon bits
PATATES COCIDOS   boiled potatoes
PATATES DORADOS   fried potatoes
PATATES FRITOS   deep fried potatoes
PATATES JUDÍAS VERDES, CON   potato and green bean
    casserole
PATATES NUEVOS   new potatoes
PATATES PAJA, DE   deep fried shoestring potatoes
PATATES PICANTES   potato slices sauteed with chili
    pepper, garlic and oil
PATATES POBRES   potato slices pan fried in garlic olive
    oil
PATATES, PURÉ DE   mashed potatoes
PATATES RELLENOS   stuffed potatoes
PATATES SALSA VERDE, CON   potato slices sauteed
    with oil, garlic and pepper
PATATES VAPOR, AL   steamed potatoes
PATÉ CAMPO, DE   country-style pâté
PATÉ CASOLANA   home-style pâté
PATÉ FOIE GRAS   goose liver pâté
PATILLA   prawn sized lobster
PATO   duck
PATO ARROZ, CON   duck and rice
PATO HORNO, AL   roast duck
PATO NABOS, CON   duck braised with turnips, onions in
    brown wine sauce
PATO NARANJA, CON   roasted duck in brown sauce,
    orange and lemon juice
PATO PERES   duck with pears

PATO PIÑA, CON   roast duck in brown sauce with
   pineapple juice
PATO RELLENO TRUFADO   roast duck stuffed with
   truffles
PATO SALVAJE ROYAL   roast wild duck
PATO SEVILLANO BRASEADO   braised duck in olive oil,
   broth, sherry, tomatoes, sliced orange
PATO SILVESTRE   wild duck
PAVO   turkey
PAVO ASADO   roast turkey
PEBRE FARCITS ANEC   sweet red pepper stuffed with
   duck
PEBRE FARCITS PORC I CALAMARS   sweet red pepper
   stuffed with pork and squid
PEBRE PIQUILLO FARCITS CON BRANDADA BACALLA
   sweet red pepper stuffed with salt cod puree
PECHO TERNERA, DE   breast of veal
PECHUGA   poultry breast
PECHUGA AVE, DE   chicken breast and wing
PECHUGA KIEV   chicken breast stuffed with butter,
   breaded and pan fried
PECHUGA NEVA   poached breast in gelatin
PECHUGA POLLO RELLENA, DE   chicken breast stuffed
   with ham, onion, wine
PECHUGA PORTUGUESA   braised chicken in tomato,
   bacon, oil
PECHUGA VILLEROI   poached chicken, breaded and
   deep fried
PEIX   fish
PELOTA   fried meat dumplings
PELOTAS   meatballs
PELOTAS COCIDAS   stew of meat wrapped in cabbage
   leaves, chicken, pork bacon, chick-peas, potatoes
PENACHO DE LEGUMBRES   mixed sauteed vegetables
PEÑASANTA   individual Baked Alaska
PEPINILLO   pickle
PEPINILLOS   gherkins, pickles

PEPINILLOS EN VINAGRE   pickled cucumbers

PEPINO   cucumber

PEPITORIA   stew with onions, green peppers and tomatoes

PEPITORIA CON GALLINA   rice and chicken fricassee
with stuffed partridge and quail, rabbit with garlic

PEPITOS   sandwich rolls

PEPITOS DE TERNERA   veal sandwich rolls

PEQUEÑA MARMITA   soup stew

PERA   pear

PERA ALMÍBAR, EN   pear in syrup

PERA BELLA ELENA   pear poached in syrup, filled with
ice cream, covered with chocolate sauce

PERAS CON VINO   stewed pears in cinnamon and wine
sauce

PERCA   perch fish

PERCEBE   barnacle

PERCEBES   goose barnacles

PERDICES AL CAPELLÁN   sauteed veal slices with ham,
salami, garlic, olive oil, wine

PERDICES ESTOFADAS   stuffed braised partridges

PERDIZ   partridge

PERDIZ BILBAÍNA   partridge braised with onion, wine,
cognac, placed on fried bread with pan juice and tomato
sauce

PERDIZ CASTELLANA   partridge braised with oil, wine,
vinegar, onion and black pepper

PERDIZ CHOCOLATE, CON   partridge in chocolate
flavored wine sauce

PERDIZ CROQUETAS COL, CON   baked partridge with
cabbage croquettes

PERDIZ ENCEBOLLADA   partridge sauteed in oil with
onions and white wine

PERDIZ ESCABECHADA   partridge braised and marinated in herb oil and vinegar

PERDIZ ESCABECHE, CON   marinated partridge

PERDIZ ESTOFADO   partridge stewed in wine, onion,
garlic

PERDIZ ESTRAGÓN, CON   partridge braised in tarragon
   sauce
PERDIZ GUISADA CON COLES   partridge stewed in
   cabbage, braised in broth, tomatoes, onions, peppers
   and oil
PERDIZ JUGO, CON   partridge roasted and served in pan
   juices
PERDIZ TOLEDANA   partridge braised in oil, vinegar,
   garlic, onions, wine
PERDIZ VINAGRETA, A LA   baked partridge in wine
   vinegar sauce
PERDIZ VINO TINTO, CON   partridge braised with oil,
   onions, garlic, tomatoes and wine
PEREJIL   parsley
PERICONA   stew containing cod, oil, dry peppers and
   garlic
PERIFOLLO   chervil
PERILLA   bland cheese
PERO   apple
PERRITOS CALIENTES   hot dogs
PESC VI I SALVIA   fish with wine and sage
PESCADILLA   fresh haddock
PESCADITO FRITO   deep-fried fish
PESCADITOS CON ESCABECHE A LA CATALANA
   fried small marinated fish with pepper and garlic
PESCADITOS CON ESCABECHE A LA ANDALUZA
   fried small marinated fish Andalusian style, with
   saffron, ginger and garlic
PESCADO   fish
PESCADO ARROZ, CON   fish and rice
PESCADO CLEOPATRA, A LA   fish boned and stuffed
   with creamed whiting paste, poached with white wine
   sauce
PESCADO FRITO GADITANA   fish fried in olive oil
PESCADO GUISADO   fish stew
PESCADO VERACRUZ   fish, Mexican style, with garlic
   and olives

PESTIÑOS   honey covered fritter

PESTIÑOS ANDALUCES   crullers with lemon and anise liqueur

PESTIÑOS CON ANÍS   licorice flavored fried pastry

PETITS FULLATS COTLLIURE   anchovy butter canapés

PETITS PASTISOS SAMFAINA ANXOVES   mixed vegetable tarts with anchovies

PETITSOUS   chocolate eclair

PEUS   feet

PEZ ESPADA   swordfish

PEZ ESPADA DE BILBAÍNA   swordfish simmered with garlic, pepper and oil

PICADA   sauce containing garlic, parsley, toasted almonds and chopped pine seeds

PICADILLA   creamy almond dressing

PICADILLO   meat mixed with diced fried potatoes; hash

PICADO   minced

PICANTE   peppery

PICATOSTE   deep-fried bread

PICHÓN   pigeon

PICHÓN CON SALSA   pigeon braised and served in onion, tomato, oil, garlic and orange juice

PICHONCILLO   squab

PICHONES   squabs *or* pigeons

PICHONES ESTOFADOS   braised stuffed squabs

PIERNA   leg

PIERNA DE CONEJO CON ALIOLI   broiled rabbit leg with garlic mayonnaise

PIERNA DE CORDERO   leg of lamb

PIERNA DE CORDERO AL HORNO   oven roasted leg of lamb

PIEZA   by the piece

PIGNOLI   pine nuts

PIJAMA   dessert with peaches, pineapple, custard, cake and ice cream

PIL-PIL   simmered

PIMENTÓN   paprika

PIMIENTO   sweet pepper

PIMIENTOS   bell peppers

PIMIENTOS CALABACINES RELLENOS   meat stuffed peppers and zucchini, baked

PIMIENTOS FRITOS   small green peppers fried in olive oil with salt

PIMIENTOS MORRÓN   red sweet peppers

PIMIENTOS MORRONES SALTEADOS   sauteed red bell peppers

PIMIENTOS RELLENOS   peppers stuffed with rice

PIMIENTOS ROJOS   red bell peppers

PIMIENTOS VERDES   green peppers

PIÑA   pineapple

PIÑA BANDA   slice of pineapple

PIÑA CONSERVA   canned pineapple

PIÑA MACERADA   crushed pineapple

PIÑA PRALINEE FLAMBÉ   pineapple with caramel, flamed

PINCHITOS CARNE   pork marinated and broiled on a skewer

PINCHO   broiled meat or mushrooms cooked on a skewer

PINCHO MORUNO   seasoned pork cubes grilled on a skewer

PIÑÓN   pine nut

PINTADA   guinea fowl

PINYÓN   pine nut

PIPARRADA   scrambled eggs with tomato, onion, ham, peppers, garlic

PIPIRRANA   salad of green pepper, onion, tomato and marinated fish

PISCO   grape brandy

PISTACHO   pistachio nut

PISTO   sauteed eggplant, green peppers and tomatoes, served cold

PISTO ARAGONÉS   salt codfish added to the vegetable mixture

PISTO BILBAÍNA, DE   ham, squash, peppers, tomatoes, onions and garlic cooked together

PISTO ESCABECHE, EN   pickled fish or meat added to the vegetable mixture

PISTO MANCHEGO   stew with red and green peppers, tomatoes, squash, onion, ham, egg or tuna added

PISTO RIOJANA, CON   stew of tomatoes, eggplant, red pepper, onion, garlic, olive oil

PIOS NONOS   chicken and potato croquettes

PIXIN   angler fish

PLANCHA   grilled

PLATAN FRITO   fried banana pastry

PLÁTANOS   bananas

PLÁTANOS CON MIEL Y PIÑONES   bananas with honey and pine nuts

PLATIJA   flounder

PLATITO   saucer

PLATO   plate

PLATO DE FRIVOLIDADES   plate of assorted pastries

PLATO DE HUEVOS   fried eggs

PLATO DE HUEVOS CHASSEUR   fried eggs in pastry shells with chicken livers and tomato-wine sauce with mushrooms

PLATO DE HUEVOS LORRENA   eggs on grilled bacon and Swiss cheese, baked

PLATO DE HUEVOS MALLORQUINA   fried eggs with sausage

PLATO DE HUEVOS MANTECA NEGRA   fried eggs with browned butter

PLATO DE HUEVOS NEGROS   fried eggs on a meat croquette with truffle sauce

PLATO DE HUEVOS ROTHMAGO   eggs on sauteed ham, baked, garnished with sausage and tomato sauce

PLATO DE HUEVOS TURBIGO   fried eggs with sausages and mushrooms or lamb kidney and grilled tomato

PLATO DE HUEVOS TURCA   fried eggs with fried onion rings, chicken livers, tomato sauce

PLATO DE HUEVOS WLADEMIR   cream coated eggs with grated cheese, browned and served with asparagus and truffles

PLATO RÉGIMEN CRUDO, DE   salad plate
PLATO TÍPICO DE LA REGIÓN   specialty of the region
PLATOS DE HOY   dishes of the day
PLATOS DEL DÍA   dishes of the day
PLATOS REGIONALES   regional dishes
POCHAS   dried white beans
POCHAS RIOJANA, CON   white beans cooked with
    garlic, onions, ham and sausage
POCHE   poached
POCO HECHO   rare
POCO PASADO   rare
POLLASTRE   chicken
POLLITO   spring chicken
POLLO   chicken
POLLO AJILLO, CON   chicken roasted with garlic
POLLO AJO, CON   chicken braised in garlic, wine, oil,
    clove and nutmeg
POLLO, ALAS DE   chicken wings in a sauce
POLLO AMERICANO   chicken breaded and grilled then
    roasted with tomatoes, bacon, fried potatoes, with sauce
    of pan juices and lemon butter; *or* split broiler with
    bread crumbs, roasted with tomatoes, French fried
    potatoes and herb butter
POLLO ASADO   roast chicken
POLLO ASADO A LA BORDELESA   chicken sauteed
    with shallots and wine
POLLO ASADO CON SALSA NARANJA   roast chicken
    with orange sauce
POLLO AST GLASEADO   chicken spit roasted with
    honey cumin glaze
POLLO CACEROLA, DE   casserole of braised chicken
    with mushrooms, carrots, bacon, peas, garlic and sherry
POLLO CASTELLANA, A LA   chicken braised in butter,
    pan juices and wine
POLLO CATALANA, A LA   chicken braised with
    eggplant, peppers, tomatoes, wine, oil
POLLO CHANFAINA   braised or stewed chicken

POLLO CHILINDRÓN   sauteed chicken with peppers, tomatoes and olives

POLLO CHILINDRÓN, CON   chicken with a tomato and pepper accompaniment

POLLO SEVILLANO, CHULETAS DE   chicken cutlets braised in tomato sauce with onions and carrots

POLLO COCOTTE   chicken braised in a casserole with butter, bacon, onions, potatoes and sherry

POLLO COCOTTE SUBAROFF   chicken stuffed with goose liver and truffles, cooked and served in sealed casserole with Madeira truffles and stock

POLLO, CRESTAS DE   cocks' crests, poached in cream sauce

POLLO ENDIABLADO   chicken basted with mustard, lemon juice, pepper flavored butter, breaded and roasted

POLLO ESCABECHE, EN   stewed marinated chicken

POLLO ESTRAGÓN   chicken roasted with vegetables and tarragon and brown tarragon sauce

POLLO FRÍO   chicken served cold

POLLO FRITO   fried chicken

POLLO FRITO GRANADINA   chicken fried in oil, garlic and wine

POLLO, GUISADO DE   stewed chicken in sauce of cinnamon, cloves, onion, wine, garlic and butter

POLLO HIGOS, CON   chicken baked with wine and figs

POLLO HORNO, AL   roast chicken with garlic and sherry

POLLO JAMONCITO, CON   boned chicken legs stuffed with mushrooms, breaded and fried

POLLO LANGOSTA, CON   chicken braised with onion, tomato, cinnamon and lobster with garlic, almonds, chestnuts, chicken liver and chocolate made into a paste

POLLO MENESTRE, CON   chicken and vegetable soup-stew

POLLO, MUSLOS DE   chicken thighs boned and stuffed with meat mixture, breaded and fried

POLLO PARRILLA, A LA   grilled chicken

POLLO PEPITORIA   chicken braised in white wine, almonds and garlic

POLLO PIBIL   chicken simmered in fruit juices

POLLO PIÑONES   sauteed chicken with pine nuts, artichokes, ham, wine

POLLO RELLENO   stuffed chicken

POLLO RELLENO PERIGOT   chicken stuffed with liver on a slice of tongue and wine sauce

POLLO RIOJANA, CON   chicken braised with tomatoes, pepper, red pepper, onion, wine

POLLO SALTEADO   sauteed chicken

POLLO SALTEADO GODARD   chicken sauteed with elaborate garnishings

POLLO SAMFAINA   chicken sauteed in wine with peppers, eggplant and tomatoes

POLLO SEVILLANA   chicken fricassee with pimentos, onion, garlic, tomato, wine, brandy and olives

POLLO VASCO   chicken braised in wine, tomatoes, peppers, mushrooms, ham, onion and garlic

POLLO VIENÉS   chicken breaded, pan fried in butter with lemon juice

POLLO VINO TINTO, CON   chicken sauteed with sausage, wine and brandy

POLVORÓN   hazelnut cookie

POLVORONES   cinnamon cookies

POLVORONES SEVILLANOS   brandy flavored butter cookies

POMELO   grapefruit

POMELO KIRSCH   grapefruit with kirsch, a cherry brandy

POMES FARCIDES   pork stuffed apples

PONCHE CON COÑAC   hot milk, almond and brandy drink

PONCHE CON CREMA   egg-nog liqueur

PONCHE SEGOVIANO   spongecake soaked in liquor with cream filling

PORCIÓN   portion

POROTOS CON GRANADOS   beans with pumpkin and corn

POROTOS NEGROS   black beans

PORTO PUDÍN Y FLAN   Portuguese baked caramel custard

PORTUGUESA   eggs cooked with tomatoes

POSTRES   desserts

POTAJE   soup; also see SOPAS

POTAJE ANDALUZ   garbanzo bean soup

POTAJE ESPINACAS Y GARBANZOS, CON   spinach, onion, chick-peas, garlic, ham

POTAJE GARBANZOS, CON   soup with garbanzo beans

POTAJE JUDÍAS BLANCAS O VERDES, CON   soup with white or green beans

POTAJE MORCILLA Y TOCINO, CON   sausage and bacon soup

POTAJE VIGILIA, DE   garbanzo beans, fish, spinach, onions, garlic, almonds, egg yolk

POTE   meat and vegetable soup-stew

POTE ASTURIANO   stew with cabbage, pig's foot, sausages, bacon, ham and white beans

POTE GALLEGO   stew with pork shoulder, white beans, potatoes, sausages, tomatoes, turnip greens, veal and chicken

POUDING   pudding

POUDING DIPLOMÁTICO   dessert with ladyfingers in liqueur, Bavarian cream or custard, apricot jam, glazed fruit soaked in rum or kirsch, and light custard sauce

POUDING FRUTAS, DE   fruit pudding

POUDING PASAS, DE   raisin pudding

POULARDA   large roasting chicken

PRALINE   roasted almonds cooked in vanilla flavored syrup, caramelized and broken into pieces

PRINCESA   eggs cooked with asparagus

PRIVADO   private

PROFITEROLES DE CHOCOLATE   pastry puffs filled with ice cream or custard, covered with chocolate sauce

PROHIBIDO EL PASO   no exit

PROHIBIDO FUMAR   no smoking

PROHIBIDO PISAR EL CÉSPED   do not walk on the grass

PROPINA   tip

PUCHERO   beef soup with vegetables

PUDÍN   pudding

PUDÍN DE MANZANA NATILLAS   apple pudding with custard sauce

PUERCO   pork

PUERCO ESTOFADO   spicy pork stew

PUERRO   leek

PULPA CON PATATINES   stewed octopus with potato, onion, garlic

PULPITOS   small octopus

PULPO   octopus

PULPO GALLEGO   octopus boiled in a sauce of paprika, pepper, garlic, olive oil

PULPO VINAGRETA, A LA   octopus boiled and marinated in wine vinegar, served cold

PULQUE   fermented drink from Mexican plant

PUNTA DE ESPÁRRAGO   asparagus tip

PUNTO   medium

PUNTO DE NIEVE   whipped cream with beaten egg whites

PURÉ   pureed *or* mashed

PURÉ GUISANTES, DE   split pea soup

PURÉ LAMBALLE   puree of pea soup and tapioca

PURÉ LEGUMBRES, DE   pureed mixed vegetable soup

PURÉ LENTEJAS, DE   pureed lentil soup with bacon and onions

PURÉ PAPAS, DE   mashed potatoes

PURÉ PARMENTIER   pureed potato soup

PURÉ PATATAS, DE   mashed potatoes

PURÉ SOLFERINO   pureed soup of tomato and potato

PURRUSALDA   dried salt codfish, leeks, potatoes, garlic made into a soup-stew

Q

QUATLLES   quail
QUEIJADAS EVORA   sweet cheese tarts
QUENELLE   dumpling of pastry and fish paste with a creamy sauce
QUESADA   sweet made with fresh cheese, honey and butter
QUESO   cheese
QUESO BANDEJA, EN   tray of assorted cheese
QUESO, CARRO DE   served from a food cart
QUESO DEL PAÍS   cheese of the area
QUESO ELEGIR   cheese of your choice
QUESO EXTRANJERO   imported cheese
QUESO GALLEGO   medium-soft cheese
QUESO, NATA DE   cream cheese
QUESO, PLATO DE   plate of cheese
QUESO, TABLA DE   a cheese board
QUESOS SURTIDOS   assorted cheeses
QUISQUILLA   very small shrimp

R

RÁBANO   radish
RÁBANO PICANTE   horse radish
RABAS   fried squid
RABO   tail
RABO DE TORO ANDALUZ   oxtail stew with wine, onion, ham
RAGÚ   stew *or* fricassee
RAJA   slice
RALLADO   grated
RANAS   frog
RAPE   firm white fish
RAPE AMERICANO   fish braised in tomato sauce made from oil, wine, onions and tomatoes
RAPE ESTILO CADAQUES   fish braised with mussels, prawns in sauce

RAPE GRELOS Y ALMEJAS, CON   fish with collard greens and clams

RAPE GRENADINA, CON   fish oven baked with sauce of garlic, onion, peppers, tomatoes, wine and olive oil

RAPE JEREZ, CON   baked white fish in sherry sauce

RAPE ORLY   battered and deep-fried white fish

RAPE RIOJANA, CON   white fish braised in oil, onion, garlic, peppers and tomato sauce

RAPE ROMESCADA   white fish braised in spicy tomato suace with oil, onion, red wine, garlic

RAVAS   bits of fried octopus

RAVIOLES   dough squares with meat or other stuffing, boiled, served with sauce and grated cheese

RAYA   skate, sea ray

REBANADA   slice

REBOZADAS   vegetables in batter, deep-fried

RECOMENDACIONES   recommendations

RECOMENDACIONES DEL CHEF   chef's recommendations

REFRESCO   soft drink

REFRITO   olive oil, parsley and garlic used to fry or sautee

REGAÑAOS   pastry with sardines and red pepper in the crust

REHOGADA   sauteed

RELÁMPAGOS   pastry similar to eclair, with filling

RELLENO   chopped meat *or* a stuffed preparation

RELLENOS   stuffed hard eggs

REMOLACHA   beetroot

REO   trout

REPOLLO   cabbage

REQUESÓN   soft, white cheese

REQUESÓN CON MIEL   cottage cheese with honey

RESERVADO   found on Chilean wine labels to indicate wine of exceptional quality

REVOLTILLO   scrambled eggs; also see HUEVOS

REVUELTOS   scrambled eggs

REVUELTOS AHUMADOS   scrambled eggs with smoked meat or fish

REVUELTOS AJETS, CON   soft scrambled eggs with scallions

REVUELTOS CALABICÍNES, CON   scrambled eggs with squash

REVUELTOS CAVIAR, CON   scrambled eggs with caviar

REVUELTOS LANGOSTINO Y ESPINACAS, CON   soft scrambled eggs with shrimp and spinach

REVUELTOS MADRILEÑOS   scrambled eggs with cream and sauteed tomatoes

REVUELTOS ORLOFF   eggs mixed with cream, crayfish and truffle added

REVUELTOS PERIGUEUX   scrambled eggs with truffle sauce

REVUELTOS VASQUERA   scrambled eggs with sauteed tomatoes and onion with Serrano ham

RIÑONES   kidneys

RIÑONES BROCHETA, EN   kidneys grilled on a skewer

RIÑONES COÑAC, CON   kidneys sauteed in sauce of pan juices and cognac

RIÑONES EN BROCHETA   veal kidneys on skewers with mushrooms, ham and bacon

RIÑONES ENSARTADOS   kidneys skewered with ham and bacon, broiled with butter

RIÑONES JEREZ, CON   kidneys in sherry wine

RIÑONES MADEIRA   kidneys sauteed with sauce from pan juices and Madeira

RIÑONES MOSTAZA, CON   kidneys sauteed in sauce from pan juices and mustard

RIÑONES PLANCHA, A LA   grilled kidneys

RIÑONES TURBIGO   kidneys sauteed on fried bread with sausages, mushrooms and pan juice, wine and tomato paste sauce

RIOJANA   fried chorizo sausage with grilled tomato

RÓBALO   haddock fish

RODABALLO   turbot, flounder-like fish

RODABALLO ARLESIANA   flounder braised in wine stock with sauce from butter, flour and fish stock, oven browned

RODABALLO CON SALSA ALBUFERA   poached
    flounder with mushroom cream sauce with bell peppers
RODAJAS   slices
ROJOES COMINO   braised pork with cumin
ROLLO DE MERLUZA   fish steak fried with ham and
    eggs in green sauce
ROMANA   dipped in batter and fried
ROMERO   rosemary
ROMESCO   sauce of olive oil, red pepper, bread, garlic,
    almonds, cognac, vinegar
RON   rum
RONCAL   spicy hard cheese made from sheep's milk
ROPA VIEJA   meat hash
ROSBIF   roast beef
ROSCAS   a cookie
ROSEXAT   saffron rice pilaf cooked in a broth with sau-
    sages and pork and bacon meatballs, browned in oven
ROSQUILLA   doughnut
ROSQUILLAS RÍO JANAS   small doughnuts made with
    wine, anise and sugar
ROSSINI   eggs with goose liver and Madeira sauce
ROVELLÓN   wild mushrooms
RUBIO   red mullet
RUIBARBO   rhubarb
RUSOS   cake with custard filling cut in squares
RUSTIDO   roast
RUSTIDO CATALANA   veal roast with rum, wine, garlic,
    pepper

S

SÁBALO   shad
SAL   salt
SALADO   salted
SALCHICHA   sausage
SALCHICHA BLANCA ASTURIANA   breakfast sausage

SALCHICHA CHABLIS, EN   sausage poached in Chablis
wine
SALCHICHA FRANKFURT   hot dog
SALCHICHA FRITA   fried sausage
SALCHICHA HIGOS AGRI-DULCES, CON   sausages
with sweet and sour figs
SALCHICHA LONGANIZA, CON   rosemary flavored
breakfast sausage
SALCHICHA RELLENA CON REPOLLO   sausage fried
in cabbage leaf
SALCHICHÓN   salami
SALCHICHÓN VICH   Catalonian sausage
SALDO   sale
SALIDO   exit
SALMI   meat in wine-liqueur sauce with fried bread
spread with meat paste
SALMÓN   salmon, fish
SALMÓN AHUMADO   smoked salmon
SALMÓN HOJALDRADO   puff pastry with salmon filling
SALMÓN RIN   Rhine salmon
SALMONETES   red mullet
SALMONETES ANDALUCES   mullets lightly battered
and deep fried
SALMONETES BERCY   mullets grilled with a white wine
sauce
SALMONETES FRANCILLÓN   mullets broiled on toast
SALMONETES GRENOBLESES   mullets pan fried with
browned butter, capers and lemon
SALMONETES MIRABEAU   mullets fried in anchovy
butter
SALMONETES PARRILLA, A LA   mullets grilled with
lemon
SALMOREJO SALSA   sauce of bread croutons, garlic, salt,
olive oil, vinegar and water ground in a mortar and pestle
SALPICÓN   tomato pulp, garlic, onions, olive oil, herbs
simmered into a tomato sauce

SALPICÓN DE AVE   chicken with mayonnaise
SALPICÓN DE MARISCOS   shrimp and lobster salad in
   tomato sauce
SALSA   sauce
SALSA ALBUFERA   mushroom flavored creamy sauce
SALSA BEARNESA   egg yolk butter sauce with wine and
   vinegar, thick and creamy
SALSA BLANCA   white sauce
SALSA CARNE   gravy
SALSA COLORADA   red sauce of tomatoes, garlic, eggs,
   almonds, olive oil, vinegar, pepper
SALSA CON SAMFAINA   sauce of oil, lard, onion, green
   peppers, eggplant, zucchini, tomatoes
SALSA DE MOSTAZA   creamy mustard-butter sauce
SALSA ESPAÑOLA   brown sauce with wine
SALSA HOLANDESA   thick sauce with lemon juice, egg
   yolks and butter
SALSA MANZANA, DE   applesauce
SALSA MAYONESA, DE   mayonnaise
SALSA MAYORDOMO, DE   butter and parsley sauce
SALSA PER CALCOTS   grilled green onion sauce
SALSA PICANTE   hot pepper sauce
SALSA ROBERT   mustard flavored meat sauce with onion
   and white wine
SALSA ROMANA   sauce of bacon or ham, egg and cream
SALSA ROMESCO   peppery sauce of tomato, hot chili
   pepper, garlic, hazelnuts, olive oil, wine vinegar
SALSA ROMESCU   red sauce of oil, vinegar, hot pepper,
   garlic, onion, pimento and tomato puree
SALSA TÁRTARA   tartar sauce
SALSA TOMATE, DE   tomato sauce
SALSA VERDE   green sauce
SALTEADO   sauteed
SALVIA   sage
SAMFAINA   half-cooked mixture of eggplant, green pep-
   per and tomato

SAN JACOBO   veal cutlet, ham slice, pork cutlet, breaded and pan-fried together

SAN SIMÓN   firm bland cheese

SANCOCHO   sama (regional fresh fish) and boiled potatoes

SANDÍA   watermelon

SANGRÍA   drink of red wine, orange liqueur and fresh fruit pieces

SANGRÍA BLANCA   drink of white wine, orange liqueur and fresh fruit pieces

SANGRITA   tequila with tomato, orange and lime juice

SARDINAS   sardines

SARDINAS ACEITE   sardines canned in oil

SARDINAS ENSARTADAS   skewered sardines

SARDINAS MONTAÑESAS   sardines boiled in grape leaves with onion, tomato, garlic, wine, mint

SCHABISCH CAUCASIANA   marinated lamb on skewer with tomato, onion, pepper and grilled

SE PROHIBE TOCAR   do not touch

SECO   dried

SEGÚN EL TAMAÑO   according to size

SELTZ   soda water

SEMIFRÍOS   frozen dessert of ice cream, candied fruits, nuts

SEMOLA   semolina

SENCILLO   plain

SENTOLLA   large crab

SEPIA   cuttlefish

SEPIONES   wild mushrooms

SEQUES   dried

SERVICIO   service

SERVICIO INCLUIDO   service included

SERVICIO NO INCLUIDO   service not included

SESOS   brains

SESOS MANTECA NEGRA, CON   brains sauteed in browned butter

SESOS MOLINERA, A LA   brains floured and fried in butter

SESOS REBOZO   brains battered and deep-fried

SESOS ROMANA, A LA   brains floured, breaded and pan-fried

SETAS   mushrooms

SETAS BORDELESA   mushrooms sauteed in olive oil, garlic, lemon juice

SEVICHE   raw fish with onions, garlic

SHANGURRO   stuffed crab

SIDRA   cider

SIERRA NEVADA   ice cream dessert covered with meringue

SOBADOS PASIEGOS   pastry rich in butter and eggs

SOBRASADA   salami; *or* spread of sausage with fat added on toast

SOBRASADA CON MALLORCA   pimiento spiced sausage from Majorca

SOFREGIT   sauce base

SOFRITO   fried sauce made with garlic, onion, tomato and parsley

SOFRITO SALSA   sauce of olive oil, onion, garlic, parsley and tomato

SOL Y SOMBRA   blend of brandy and aniseed liqueur

SOLLA   plaice *or* flounder

SOLO   straight

SOLOMILLO   filet *or* entrecote

SOLOMILLO ALL PEBRE   beef roast in a pepper garlic sauce

SOLOMILLO CASADOR   filet sauteed in butter in sauce of pan juices, wine, mushrooms

SOLOMILLO DIPLOMÁTICO   whole filet, larded, marinated in wine, pan roasted and served with a sauce from pan juices and wine

SOLOMILLO ESPAÑOL   larded whole filet, pan fried in oil with a sherry gravy with onion, garlic, and oregano

SOLOMILLO HORTELANO   filet sauteed in earthenware
pot in sauce from pan juices and butter

SOLOMILLO MAÎTRE D'HÔTEL   grilled steaks with
creamed butter and lemon juice

SOLOMILLO PARRILLA, A LA   charcoal broiled steaks

SOLOMILLO PIEMONTESE   fried steak in tomato sauce
with pan juices

SOLOMILLO PRUSIANA   steak on charcoal broiler

SOLOMILLO WELLINGTON   whole tenderloin covered
with sauteed mushrooms and cooked vegetables in
pastry dough

SOPA   soup; also see CREMAS, CONSOMES

SOPA AJO Y HUEVO, DE   garlic soup with egg

SOPA AJO Y PESCADO, DE   garlic soup with fish stock

SOPA AJO, DE   garlic soup with eggs

SOPA ALBÓNDIGAS, DE   meatballs of veal and chicken
in chicken broth

SOPA ALENTEJANA   coriander and garlic soup with
poached eggs

SOPA ANCAS DE RANA, DE   frog's legs soup

SOPA ARROZ, DE   rice cooked in bouillon with chicken
livers, vegetables or meats

SOPA BOLETS, DE   mushroom soup

SOPA CANTÁBRICA   fish soup

SOPA CASTELLANA   bread, preferably the broth of a
stew, ham, sometimes a poached egg and garlic

SOPA CEBOLLA, DE   onion soup

SOPA CLARA   clear soup

SOPA COCIDA   soup part of soup-stew, with rice or pasta

SOPA CODA BUEY, DE   oxtail soup

SOPA COLA DE BUEY, DE   oxtail soup

SOPA CREMA, DE   cream of chicken soup

SOPA CUARTO DE HORA, DE   soup with olive oil, shrimp,
ham, peas, tomatoes, onion, clams, boiled egg, rice

SOPA DE ALMENDRAS Y CEBOLLA   onion and almond
soup

SOPA DEL DÍA   soup of the day
SOPA ESPAÑOLA   spiced soup with rice, tomatoes and
   peppers
SOPA ESPESA   thick soup
SOPA FIDEOS, DE   soup with noodles or pasta
SOPA FREDOLICS   wild mushroom soup
SOPA GALLINA CON PASTA, DE   chicken noodle soup
SOPA GARBANZOS Y CHORIZO, DE   chick-peas,
   sausage, garlic, pepper and bacon soup
SOPA GUISANTES, DE   pea soup
SOPA IMPERIAL   chicken and veal broth thickened with
   tapioca, with sherry and cubes of wine-flavored custard;
   cream of rice and tapioca soup; consommé with egg
   yolks and ham
SOPA JAMÓN, CON   soup with ham
SOPA JULIANA   vegetable soup with garlic
SOPA LANGOSTA, DE   spiny lobster soup
SOPA LEGUMBRES, DE   vegetable soup
SOPA LENTEJAS, DE   lentil soup
SOPA MALAGUEÑA   seafood soup with saffron, absinthe
   liquor, egg yolks, croutons
SOPA MARINERA   seafood soup
SOPA MARISCOS, DE   seafood soup
SOPA MARISQUERA   seafood soup
SOPA MEJILLONES, DE   mussel soup
SOPA MENUDO, DE   chicken giblet soup
SOPA MERLUZA, DE   hake fish soup
SOPA MOSCOVITA   milk and egg based soup with nut-
   meg seasoning
SOPA PANELA, DE   garlic soup with chick-peas, mint
   and croutons
SOPA PASTA, DE   soup with pasta
SOPA PATATAS, DE   potato soup
SOPA PAVESA   beef broth poured over toasted bread
   topped with raw egg and grated cheese, then browned
SOPA PESCADO CATALÁN, DE   fish soup with shellfish,
   fish, onion, tomato, olive oil, garlic

SOPA PESCADO GADITANA, DE   fish soup with garlic, onion, orange juice

SOPA PESCADO VASCA   fish soup with mussels, carrots, onion, shallots, olive oil, cognac, butter

SOPA PESCADO, DE   fish soup

SOPA PESCADORES   fish soup

SOPA PICADILLO, DE   thick soup with chicken, veal or ham, with beaten egg poured into hot soup before serving

SOPA PICANTE   goulash soup

SOPA PUCHERO, DE   beef soup

SOPA QUESO, DE   soup with cheese

SOPA RABO DE BUEY, DE   oxtail soup with vegetables and wine

SOPA RAPE, DE   fish soup with onions, garlic, tomato, celery, bread, vinegar, nuts and spices

SOPA REAL   clear broth with pastries or dumplings

SOPA SEVILLANA   highly seasoned fish soup

SOPA TOMATE, DE   tomato soup

SOPA TORTUGA, DE   turtle-rice soup

SOPA TRUCHA, DE   trout soup

SOPA TURBOT Y GAMBAS, DE   fish and prawn soup

SOPA VERDURAS, DE   vegetable soup

SOPA VIGILIA, DE   shellfish and fish soup with vegetables, sherry and hard-boiled egg

SORBETE   iced fruit drink

SORBETE DE CHAMPÁN   champagne sherbet

SORBETE DE TURRÓN   ice milk made with almonds and honey

SOUFFLÉ   baked egg dish with various flavorings or grated ingredients

SOUFFLÉ DE SALMÓN   baked egg dish with salmon

SOUFFLÉ DE SESOS   baked egg dish with sauteed brains

SOUFFLÉ DE ZANAHORIAS   baked egg dish with carrots

SPAGETTIS   spaghetti

SPAGETTIS A LA BOLOÑESA   spaghetti with meat and vegetable sauce

SPAGETTIS A LA INGLESA   spaghetti with veal gravy,
    grated Parmesan cheese, baked
SPAGETTIS BILBAÍNA   cooked spaghetti with crabmeat
    in a tomato sauce with onion, garlic, broth and paprika
SPAGETTIS ITALIANOS   spaghetti with butter and
    grated cheeses
SPAGETTIS NAPOLITANOS   spaghetti with tomato sauce,
    garlic and onion sauteed in olive oil with grated cheese
STEAK DIANA   pan fried steak in creamy pepper sauce
STEAK TARTAR   raw ground beef with raw egg, chopped
    onions and capers
SU PUNTO   medium
SUAVE   soft
SUCULENTO   corn, squash and other vegetables
SUFLÉ   soufflé
SUGERENCIAS DEL CHEF   chef's suggestions
SUIZO   bun
SUIZOS   baked sugar topped breakfast sweet rolls
SULTANAS   raisins
SUQUET   fish stew-soup of clams, mussels, garlic,
    almonds, fish broth
SUQUILLO DE PESCADORES   fish soup-stew
SURTIDO   assorted
SURTIDOS FIAMBRES   cold meat slices
SYRUP GRANADINA   pomegranate syrup mixed in wine
    or brandy

T

TABLA   cheese board
TABURETE   steak fried in olive oil
TACO   cornmeal or wheat pancake with meat or chicken
    filling, served with a spicy sauce
TAJADA   slice
TAJADA DE ESTOFADO   fricassee
TAJADA DE FILETE   filet
TAJADA DE HÍGADO   liver

TAJADA DE PICADILLO   knuckle
TAJADA DE RIÑÓN   kidneys
TAJADA DE SESOS   brains
TALLARINES   noodles
TALLARINES CATALANOS   noodles in sauce with pork spare ribs, sausage, onion, tomato, garlic, almonds
TALLINA   clam or mussel stew
TALLINA CATALANA   clams in tomato garlic sauce
TAMAL   pastry dough with meat or fruit filling, steamed in corn husks
TAMALES   ground meat rolled in cornmeal dough
TAMALES CALIENTES   hot tamales
TAPA   appetizer
TAPAS CABRALE Y PIÑONES   blue cheese and pine nut spread on toast
TAPAS DE ANCHOA Y PIMIENTO   anchovy and pimento spread on toast
TARDE   afternoon
TARTA   tart *or* pie
TARTA ALMENDRAS, DE   almond cake
TARTA CAPUCHINA   sponge cake with custard topping
TARTA CIRUELAS, DE   plums layered with cookies or sponge cake, sprinkled with liquor
TARTA CONVENTO, DE   puff pastry tart with chocolate glaze
TARTA GALLEGA   almond cake
TARTA HELADA   ice cream tart
TARTA HUERTO CURA, DEL   cake with frozen orange custard and orange liqueur
TARTA MANTEQUILLA, DE   cookies or spongecake spread with a chocolate butter cream filling, meringue, nuts and fruits
TARTA MANZANA, DE   open face apple cake with custard inside
TARTA MIL HOJAS   Napoleon
TARTA NARANJA, CON   orange almond cake with orange syrup

TARTA NORMANDA   made with apples

TARTA NUECES, CON   chocolate cake with chopped nuts

TARTA PIÑONES, CON   tart with pine nuts

TARTA PONCHE, CON   layered cake with cream filling and chopped almonds

TARTA QUESO, DE   cheesecake

TARTA SANTIAGO   almond cake with almond topping

TARTA YEMAS, CON   cake with liquor soaked sponge-cake

TARTELETAS   pastry crust filled with cream sauce mixture of seafood, chicken or meat

TARTALETAS CON CHAMPIÑÓN   pastry tarts filled with mushrooms

TARTALETAS CON SALMÓN   pastry tarts filled with salmon

TARTINA   slice of buttered bread topped with a filling

TAZA   soup served in a cup

TAZA DE CAFÉ   cup of coffee

TÉ   tea

TECLA CON YEMA   baked puff pastry horns with candied egg yolk filling

TENCA   tench, fresh water fish

TEQUILA   brandy made from aloe plant

TERNASCO   baby lamb

TERNASCO ASADO   roasted baby lamb

TERNASCO ASADO ARAGONÉS   baby lamb roasted over coals

TERNASCO, CABEZA ASADA DE   roasted baby lamb's head

TERNASCO, COSTILLAS DE   baby lamb chops

TERNASCO PASTORA, A LA   baby lamb braised in pepper, clove, garlic, vinegar and white wine, milk, oil and potatoes

TERNERA   veal

TERNERA ASADA   oven roasted veal leg

TERNERA BRASEADA   roast veal with pan juice and tomato sauce, with spinach cakes

TERNERA, CABEZA DE   boned and poached veal head

TERNERA, CALDERETA DE   potted roast veal leg

TERNERA CHOP INGLESA   breaded veal chops fried in butter

TERNERA CON BLANQUETA   veal stew in white herb gravy

TERNERA CONDESITA   veal with sherry

TERNERA EN AGUJA   veal in baked pastry

TERNERA, ESCALOPE DE   veal cutlet

TERNERA ESTOFADA   veal stew

TERNERA EXTREMEÑA   sauteed veal with sausage, green peppers, sherry

TERNERA, FALDA DE   veal flank steak

TERNERA EMPANADOS, FILETES DE   breaded cutlets pan fried in olive oil

TERNERA CATALÁN, FRICOANDO DE   stew with onion, tomato, mushrooms and wine

TERNERA GRANADINAS, CON   thick veal cutlets of top round larded with pork fat

TERNERA GUISADA   stewed veal

TERNERA GUISANTES, CON   roast veal with green peas

TERNERA HIGADO, CON   veal liver

TERNERA JARDINERA   roasted veal with cooked fresh vegetables and a sauce of pan juices and pureed vegetables

TERNERA, LENGUA DE   veal tongue slices

TERNERA MADRILEÑA   ham slice between two veal cutlets that are floured and pan fried

TERNERA, MANO DE   calf's foot

TERNERA MECHADA   veal larded with pork, bacon fat or ham

TERNERA MEDALLÓN VICTORIA   sauteed meat served on a chicken croquette with fried tomato

TERNERA MENESTRA, Y   veal and vegetable soup-stew

TERNERA, MOLLEJAS DE   sweetbreads

TERNERA MORCILLO   veal shank

TERNERA PASTEL   veal pâté

TERNERA, PECHO DE   roasted, stuffed and rolled breast
of veal

TERNERA, PEZ DE   bottom round veal

TERNERA, PICADILLO DE   veal hash

TERNERA, PINCHOS DE   veal cubes, marinated,
skewered and grilled

TERNERA, PULPETAS DE   veal cutlets with a meat paste
spread, rolled, breaded and fried

TERNERA REDONDO ASADO   bottom round roast veal

TERNERA RIOJANA, CON   stew with wine, lard, bacon
and pigs' feet with tomato puree

TERNERA, ROLLO DE   breaded veal loaf with ham,
onion, almond paste, oven-braised

TERNERA SALTEADA CASERA   veal braised with wine
and vegetables in brown tomato gravy

TERNERA SEVILLANA   sauteed veal with sherry

TERNERA, SOLOMILLO DE   tenderloin steak

TERNERA TRUFADA   loin spread with veal paste, bacon,
ham, truffles, rolled up and poached

TERNERA, ZANCARRÓN DE   braised veal foot

TERRINA   meat or fish paste usually in pastry shell

TERRINA DE CONEJO   rabbit pâté

TERRINA DE PERDIZ   partridge and liver pâté

TESTÍCULOS TORO ALLI I JULIVERT   bull's testicles
with garlic and parsley

TIEMPO   in season

TINTO   red wine

TÍO PEPE   a brand name for sherry

TOCINILLO CIELLO   sweet made with egg yolk and sugar

TOCINO   bacon

TOCINO DE CIELO   rich caramel custard with syrup inside

TOJUNTO   rabbit, garlic, onion, green pepper, olive oil all
cooked together

TOMATES   tomatoes

TOMATES PROVENZAL   tomatoes with garlic flavored
   crum stuffing, baked
TOMATES RELLENOS RIA AROSA   tomatoes stuffed
   with shrimp, clams, onions, wine, cognac
TOMILLO   thyme
TONYINA   tuna
TORDO   thrush
TORO   bull
TORO, COLA DE   tail
TORO LIDIA   fighting bull
TORO, RABO DE   tail
TORONJA   grapefruit
TORRIJAS   French toast
TORRIJAS CON VINO   wine-dipped French toast
TORTA   pancake
TORTA ARROZ LECHE, DE   rice pudding cake
TORTA CHICHARRONES, CON   baked bread with
   crunchy pork fat pieces, sugar, egg and lemon rind
TORTA MOCA, DE   mocha layer cake with rum
TORTAS ACEITE, CON   anise and sesame seed cookies
TORTAS CARNE, DE   meat patties
TORTELES   baked, almond paste filled, sweet bread rings
TORTERA   pastry
TORTILLA   omelette plain or with cheese, ham, mush-
   rooms, chicken livers, seafood filling; also see HUEVOS
TORTILLA ABUELO   omelette with parsley and fried
   bread cubes
TORTILLA AJITOS SILVESTRES, CON   omelette with
   young, wild garlic
TORTILLA ALICANTINA   omelette with onion, shrimp,
   asparagus, ham and tomato
TORTILLA AMPURDANESA   omelette with cooked
   white beans
TORTILLA ANDALUZA   omelette with sauteed
   tomatoes, ham, pimiento, mushrooms
TORTILLA ANGUILAS, CON   omelette with fried baby eels
TORTILLA ARANJUEZ   omelette with asparagus tips

TORTILLA ASTURIANA   omelette with tuna fish, onion and tomato

TORTILLA ATÚN ESCABECHADO, DE   omelette with marinated tuna fish and onion

TORTILLA ATÚN, DE   omelette with potatoes, spinach, chunks of tuna

TORTILLA BACALAO, DE   omelette with codfish and onion

TORTILLA BETANZOS   potato omelette

TORTILLA BUENA MUJER   fried bacon, fried onion and mushroom omelette

TORTILLA CATALANA   omelette with sauteed tomatoes, green pepper and eggplant

TORTILLA CHAMPIÑONES, CON   omelette with mushroom, ham, garlic

TORTILLA CHANGET   omelette with fried whitebait fish

TORTILLA CHORIZO, CON   omelette with spicy sausage

TORTILLA COMBINADA   omelette with combination of local ingredients

TORTILLA CONFITURA, CON   jam omelette

TORTILLA CORUÑESA   omelette with potatoes and cured ham

TORTILLA DÁTILES, CON   omelette with shrimp, ham, dates, tomato sauce

TORTILLA DE GRANADA   omelette made with lamb sweetbreads, chicken liver and kidney with white wine

TORTILLA DE SU ELECCIÓN   omelette of your choice

TORTILLA DULCE   jam omelette

TORTILLA ESCABECHE, CON   omelette with pickled fish

TORTILLA ESPAÑOLA   omelette with sliced potatoes and onions fried in oil

TORTILLA ESTRAGÓN, CON   omelette with tarragon

TORTILLA EXTREMEÑA   omelette with sausage and potatoes

TORTILLA FINES DE HIERBAS, CON   omelette with chopped fresh herbs

TORTILLA FRANCESA   plain tortilla

TORTILLA GALLEGA   omelette with potatoes, ham, red
sweet peppers and peas

TORTILLA GAMBAS, CON   omelette with prawns and
prawn sauce

TORTILLA GARBANZOS, CON   omelette with chick-peas

TORTILLA HABAS, CON   omelette with lima beans

TORTILLA HÚNGARA   omelette with onions sauteed
with ham and paprika cream sauce

TORTILLA JAMÓN, DE   ham omelette

TORTILLA JARDINERA   omelette with mixed vegetables

TORTILLA LACÓN, CON   omelette with pork shoulder
meat

TORTILLA LEGUMBRES, CON   omelette with mixed,
diced, cooked vegetables

TORTILLA LORRENA   omelette with grilled bacon,
Gruyere cheese, cream and chives mixed in eggs

TORTILLA LYONESA   omelette with sliced fried onions
and eggs

TORTILLA MAGRA   lean ham omelette

TORTILLA MARINESCA   seafood omelette

TORTILLA MURCIANA   omelette with sauteed tomatoes,
onions, squash, eggplant

TORTILLA NAVARRA   tomatoes sauteed with garlic,
eggs on top, with fried sausage, cheese, oven-baked

TORTILLA PAISANA   omelette with ham and vegetables

TORTILLA PATATA ESPAÑOLA, DE   Spanish potato
omelette

TORTILLA PATATAS, DE   omelette made with potatoes
and onions, fried in olive oil

TORTILLA SABOYARDA   eggs mixed with Swiss cheese
and poured over sauteed potatoes

TORTILLA SACROMONTE   omelette made with fried
and breaded brain, lamb or veal testicles, potatoes, red
pepper and peas

TORTILLA SESOS, CON   omelette with sauteed brains

TORTILLA SETAS, CON   omelette with wild mushrooms

TORTILLITAS CON CAMARONES   shrimp pancakes

TORTITA   waffle

TORTUGA   turtle

TOSTADA   toast

TOSTADAS   French toast with honey

TOSTADO   toast

TOSTÓN   spit roasted young suckling pig

TOUCINHO CEU   almond cake

TOURNEDOS   steak from middle of the filet

TOURNEDOS ALEXANDRA   steak sauteed with sliced truffles

TOURNEDOS BAYANA   steak pan fried and covered with tomato sauce

TOURNEDOS BEATRIX   steak pan fried with sauteed morel mushrooms, artichoke hearts, potatoes, with brown meat sauce

TOURNEDOS BILBAÍNA   steak marinated in oil with garlic paste, breaded and broiled

TOURNEDOS BOUQUETIERE   steak grilled with fresh vegetables

TOURNEDOS BRUXELLOISE   steak pan fried in butter with Madeira sauce from pan juices, served with Brussels sprouts, endive and potatoes

TOURNEDOS CASADOROS   steak pan fried in brown wine sauce with mushrooms, shallots and tomato paste

TOURNEDOS COSTA VASCA, DE   steak sauteed and topped with tomatoes

TOURNEDOS EMPERADOR, AL   steak pan fried with truffle, Madeira sauce

TOURNEDOS ENRIQUE IV, AL   steak pan fried on fried bread with artichoke bottom stuffed with butter, wine and tarragon sauce

TOURNEDOS ESPAÑOLES   steak pan fried with fried sliced onions, grilled tomatoes, rice pilaf with peppers

TOURNEDOS FAVORITOS   steak sauteed with goose liver and truffle

TOURNEDOS FINANCIEROS   steak pan fried with brown meat sauce

TOURNEDOS MARISCALA, A LA   steak sauteed and topped with truffle with concentrated meat gelatin glaze

TOURNEDOS MASCOTA, A LA   steak sauteed in earthenware with brown sauce from pan juices, wine and veal gravy

TOURNEDOS POMPADOUR, A LA   steak sauteed with truffle slice, truffle flavored brown sauce

TOURNEDOS RICHELIEU   pan fried or grilled steak

TOURNEDOS ROSSINI   steak pan fried in butter, laid on fried bread with slice of fried goose liver, with Madeira and pan juice sauce

TREMPO   salad

TRIPAS   tripe, stomach lining of a cow

TRIPAS CATALANA   tripe stewed with wine, tomato, pine nuts, almonds, garlic

TRIPAS PORTO   tripe stew

TRIPLE SECO   orange liqueur

TRONCO   slice of

TROUXA VITELA   veal roast with red onion

TRUCHA   trout

TRUCHA ALMENDRAS, CON   trout fried in butter with sliced almonds and browned butter

TRUCHA ASTURIANA   trout pan fried with bacon and tomato, paprika, lemon sauce

TRUCHA CREMA, CON   trout oven simmered in shallot, garlic, wine and cream sauce

TRUCHA ESCABECHADA   marinated trout, served cold

TRUCHA FILIPE V   fried trout and bacon, on milk soaked bread, covered with orange slices on cooked cabbage and oven baked

TRUCHA FRITA ASTURIANA   trout fried in butter

TRUCHA NAVARRA   pan fried trout stuffed with ham

TRUCHA SARTÉN, DE   trout sauteed in butter and oil

TRUCHA SEGOVIANA   trout fried in olive oil, with sauce of garlic, ham and lemon

TRUCHA WHISKEY   trout pan fried in butter, flamed with whiskey

TRUFAS   truffles, a fungus grown underneath the ground
TRUITA DE PATATA   potato omelette
TRUITA SAMFAINA   mixed vegetable omelette
TUÉTANO TOSTADA   bone marrow poached and served
   on fried bread
TUMBET   cake of potato and fried eggplant, covered with
   tomato sauce and peppers, then boiled
TURBO   turbot
TURCA   with chicken livers
TURRÓN   whole almonds mixed with honey and sugar
TURRÓN ALICANTE   hard white almond nougat
TURRONES   almond paste

U

ULLOA   soft cheese like camembert
UMA SALADA PORTUGUESA   mixed green salad
URTA   sea bass fish *or* porgy
URTA ROTENA   baked porgy and peppers with brandy
URTA SAL   porgy baked in salt accompanied with sauce
UVA   grape
UVA PASA   raisin

V

VACA   beef
VACA SALADA   corned beef
VAINILLA   vanilla
VALENCIANA   with rice, tomatoes and garlic
VARIADO   assorted
VARIOS   sundries
VARIOS AROMAS   various flavors
VASO   glass
VASO DE AGUA   glass of water
VASO DE LECHE   glass of milk
VEDELLA   veal

VEIRAS GRATINADAS   baked scallops in wine
VELDELLA PERES   roast veal loin with pears
VENADO   venison
VENERA   scallop
VENTRESCA ACEITE   belly meat of tuna in olive oil
VERDURAS   vegetables
VERMICELLI   thin spaghetti
VERMUT   vermouth
VETERANO OSBORNE   wine distilled brandy
VICHYSSOISE   chilled, creamed leek and potato soup
VIEIRAS   scallops in the shell, with pepper, onions,
    parsley and bread crumbs, put into the oven
VIEIRAS GALLEGAS   scallops braised in onion sauce
    with garlic, peppers and wine
VIEIRAS SAN JACOBO   scallops on the half-shell, in a
    thick tomato sauce, served oven browned
VIEIRAS SANTIAGO   baked scallops with brandy and
    wine in shells
VILLAGODIO DE VACA   large rib steak of beef
VILLALÓN   cheese from sheep's milk
VINAGRE   vinegar
VINAGRETA   oil and vinegar salad dressing
VINO   wine
VINO BLANCO   white wine
VINO BURDEOS   bordeaux
VINO CLARETE   rosé wine
VINO COMÚN   table wine
VINO CORRIENTE   local wine
VINO DE LA REGIÓN   local wine
VINO DE MESA   table wine
VINO DEL PAÍS   local wine
VINO DULCE   dessert wine
VINO ESPUMOSO   sparkling wine
VINO ROSADO   rosé wine
VINO SECO   dry wine
VINO SUAVE   sweet wine

VINO TINTO   red wine
VIVAS   raw oysters on the half shell
VIZCAÍNA   with green peppers, tomatoes, garlic

X

XAI   lamb
XAMPÁÑ   sparkling wine
XATO   peppery salad of curly endive with meats and
  sausages
XOCOLATA   chocolate

Y

YAUTIA   sweet potato
YEMAS   whipped egg yolks and sugar
YEMAS COCO   coconut candies made with brandy
YERBA MATE   South American holly tea
YOGHOURT   yogurt

Z

ZABAGLIONE   soft custard of cooked beaten egg yolks,
  sugar and wine
ZAMBURIÑA   a scallop
ZANAHORIAS   carrots
ZANAHORIAS GLASEADAS   carrots glazed with butter
  and sugar
ZANAHORIAS VICHY   carrots glazed with butter and
  sugar with Vichy water
ZANCARRÓN VASCO   braised veal foot with ham, sliced
  sausage, fried onions, peppers, tomatoes and broth
ZARZAMORA   blackberry
ZARZUELA   seafood chowder *or* stew
ZARZUELA DE PESCADO   fish with seasoned sauce
ZARZUELA DE VERDURAS   vegetable stew
ZORZA   chorizo sausage meat

ZUMO   juice
ZUMO FRUTA   fruit juice
ZUMO LIMÓN   lemon juice
ZUMO NARANJA   orange juice
ZUMO POMELO   grapefruit juice
ZURRACAPOTE   stewed apricots and prunes